Communication Studies and Feminist Perspectives on Ovarian Cancer

Lexington Studies in Health Communication

Series Editors: Leandra H. Hernández and Kari Nixon

National and international governments have recognized the importance of widespread, timely, and effective health communication, as research shows that accurate, patient-centered, and culturally competent health communication can improve patient and community health care outcomes. This interdisciplinary series examines the role of health communication in society and is receptive to manuscripts and edited volumes that use a variety of theoretical, methodological, interdisciplinary, and intersectional approaches. We invite contributions on a variety of health communication topics including but not limited to health communication in a digital age; race, gender, ethnicity, class, physical abilities, and health communication; critical approaches to health communication; feminisms and health communication; LGBTQIA health; interpersonal health communication perspectives; rhetorical approaches to health communication; organizational approaches to health communication; health campaigns, media effects, and health communication; multicultural approaches to health communication; and international health communication. This series is open to contributions from scholars representing communication, women's and gender studies, public health, health education, discursive analyses of medical rhetoric, and other disciplines whose work interrogates and explores these topics. Successful proposals will be accessible to an interdisciplinary audience, advance our understanding of contemporary approaches to health communication, and enrich our conversations about the importance of health communication in today's health landscape.

Recent Titles in This Series

Communication Studies and Feminist Perspectives on Ovarian Cancer, by Dinah A. Tetteh

Reifying Women's Experiences with Invisible Illness: Illusions, Delusions, Reality, edited by Kesha Morant Williams and Frances Selena Morant

Communication Studies and Feminist Perspectives on Ovarian Cancer

Dinah A. Tetteh

LEXINGTON BOOKS
Lanham • Boulder • New York • London

Published by Lexington Books
An imprint of The Rowman & Littlefield Publishing Group, Inc.
4501 Forbes Boulevard, Suite 200, Lanham, Maryland 20706
www.rowman.com

Unit A, Whitacre Mews, 26-34 Stannary Street, London SE11 4AB

Chapter 5 is an Author's Original Manuscript of an article published by Taylor & Francis Group in *Women's Reproductive Health* on March 21, 2017, available online DOI: 10.1080/23293691.2017.1276371.

British Library Cataloguing in Publication Information Available

Library of Congress Cataloging-in-Publication Data

Names: Tetteh, Dinah A., author.
Title: Communication studies and feminist perspectives on ovarian cancer / Dinah A. Tetteh.
Description: Lanham : Lexington Books, [2017] | Series: Lexington studies in health communication | Includes bibliographical references and index.
Identifiers: LCCN 2018000937 (print) | LCCN 2017061500 (ebook) | ISBN 9781498548120 (electronic) | ISBN 9781498548113 (cloth : alk. paper)
Subjects: LCSH: Ovaries--Tumors. | Ovaries--Cancer.
Classification: LCC RC280.O8 (print) | LCC RC280.O8 T43 2017 (ebook) | DDC 616.99/465--dc23
LC record available at https://lccn.loc.gov/2018000937

∞™ The paper used in this publication meets the minimum requirements of American National Standard for Information Sciences Permanence of Paper for Printed Library Materials, ANSI/NISO Z39.48-1992.

Printed in the United States of America

Contents

Acknowledgments

This book developed out of a study I conducted with ovarian cancer survivors in northwest Ohio and southern Michigan. I am grateful to the survivors for their time and willingness to make bare some of the darkest moments of their lives. Some of them were living with recurrent disease and/or were about to begin treatments due to recurrences—they were fighting for their lives—yet made time to talk with me. Thank you! My immense appreciation also goes to Gini Steinke, founder and executive director of Ovarian Cancer Connection in Toledo, Ohio, and Jean Schoen, founder of Cancer Connection of Northwest Ohio, for their support of this project.

A heartfelt thank you to Dr. Sandra Faulkner, my mentor and advisor, for encouraging me to write this book. Thank you for being an example of all that is possible, for proving that writing can become a habit, for selflessly investing in my growth as a scholar, and for carefully reading and providing feedback on earlier drafts of this book. I also thank Dr. Radhika Gajjala for the continued mentorship and support, and Dr. Lisa Hanasono for your inspiring disposition. I am also grateful for the support of colleagues in the Department of Communication at Arkansas State University, especially Dr. Marcie Hayes.

I would like to acknowledge the love, support, and prayers of my family in Ghana and the United States. My gratitude to my partner, Ernest Amanor-Opata, for the encouragement and love. And, I thank my spiritual parents, Dr. Arnold Nyarambi and Pastor Dumisa Nyarambi, for being my life coaches and teaching me to prize professionalism, diligence, and humility. For their support and friendship, I thank Mariam and Alex Kamasah, Dr. Barnabas Otoo, Tio Sitambuli, Edmund Adem, Fang Wang, Zehui Dai, and Shrinkhala Upadhyaya.

Research for this book was supported by a non-service dissertation fellowship grant (2015–16) I received from the School of Media and Communication at Bowling Green State University.

Chapter One

Introduction

In 2013 and 2015, Oscar-winning US actress and director, Angelina Jolie, disclosed in opinion editorials in *The New York Times* that she had a double mastectomy and oophorectomy (i.e., removal of the ovaries) as preventative treatments for cancer because of faulty BRCA1 gene and family history of cancer. Jolie explained her gene mutation placed her at 87 percent chance of getting breast cancer and 50 percent chance of having ovarian cancer; the double mastectomy reduced her risk of breast cancer to under 5 percent (Jolie, 2013). Her 2013 announcement created what has come to be known as "Angelina Jolie effect" where many women were inspired to consider genetic testing to determine their risks of cancer (Kluger & Park, 2013; Sunnybrooks Health Sciences Center, 2014; "The Angelina Jolie Effect," 2013). Jolie explained in the 2015 editorial that the decision to remove her ovaries and fallopian tubes (in a procedure called laparoscopic bilateral salpingo-oophorectomy) was tough and that she felt "feminine" and confident that "my children will never have to say, "Mom died of ovarian cancer" (Jolie, 2015, p. 15). Jolie was hailed by sections of the public as brave, courageous, and as setting an example for women; some also described her announcements as "feminist victory" (Dean, 2016; Kaplan, 2015, p. 14; Kluger & Park, 2013; Michel, 2014).

As I argued elsewhere, Jolie's medical announcements help explicate how some women's health issues get credence and visibility than others and how ovarian cancer is supposedly invisible not only because the ovaries are in the interior of the female body or because the disease sometimes presents nonspecific symptoms. Ovarian cancer is *made* invisible by cultural perceptions of the ovary and by system policies and politics, including eligibility criteria for treating risk of hereditary breast and ovarian cancer (HBOC) and health insurance policies for funding predictive testing and preventative treatments for at-risk women. Further, Jolie's case underscores complexities and limitations of "choice" and "risk" touted in women's health (Happe, 2013, 2017; Lippman, 1999), and demonstrates how rhetoric of risk impacts women's embodiment of risk and management practices, including removal of healthy body parts (e.g., breasts and ovaries; Happe, 2006). Her case provides a current example of the link between social constructions of the ovary (as defective and relevant only for reproductive purposes) and perspectives about genomics and genetic testing, helping reify how genomics "reaffirms the place of the ovary (and the women tied to it) in the social and economic order" (Happe, 2013, p. 179). Jolie does not have ovarian cancer or breast cancer but is at risk; she is a previvor.

Importantly, Jolie's case provides context (from popular culture perspective) for arguments in this book, including invisibility of ovarian cancer, prevailing views about diseased female body parts (e.g., breasts and ovaries), and presumed roles reconstructive surgery plays in masking harms cancer treatments inflict on the feminine body. This book argues that values attached to the female body and notions about which parts are essential and unessential to femininity impact women's interpretations of effects of ovarian cancer treatments on their sexual self-concepts, including actions taken to protect sense of self and relational others (e.g., wearing scarves, wigs, and makeup). Traditional feminine beauty standards upheld by the social environments women[1] inhibit become part of available frameworks to interpret effects of treatments on their physical, relational, and psychological selves. These standards intersect with demographic variables and disease characteristics to determine younger and older survivors' communicative responses to effects of treatments. I contend that societal standards and demands of beauty rob women of the agency to fully embody their cancer experiences. On the other hand, women's embodiments of effects of treatments also challenge normative views about feminine beauty, possibly helping explain why society shies away from the disease. This book argues that it is in the image of a sick, scarred, and worn-out body that ovarian cancer survivors are certain they are well and/or getting rid of the disease. It is when women look sick with no hair, that they are assured they are actually well and healthy. While this points to implications of cultural meanings of suffering for cancer survivors' perceptions about effectiveness of treatments (Bell, 2009), it also suggests a need for critical engagements with meanings of the embodied ovarian cancer experience.

Further, Jolie's preventative mastectomy announcement provides visible reinforcement of the 'survival' and 'proactive' rhetoric of cancer and the media highlighted this to prove that women can in fact embrace their health challenges without any harm to the feminine body. Popular cancer awareness discourses encourage women to be proactive about their own health (and know their bodies) to enhance early detection of disease. The "war on cancer" metaphor presumes that with the appropriate tests and treatments (and the right attitude by the patient) the war can be won and women can return to 'normal' life (Dubriwny, 2009; Macilwain, 2015). Jolie's situation highlights the perception that control over breast cancer is somewhat in the hands of women whereas ovarian cancer is still a medical puzzle. Thus, the public can safely engage in discussions about breast cancer but ovarian cancer is hardly broached because lay people supposedly lack the expertise and resources to get a handle on the disease. As I will show, however, the 'proactive' and early diagnosis rhetoric of cancer is problematic as it erroneously constructs an identity of cancer survivorship and obscures attention to larger societal problems, including inequalities in the health care system (King, 2006). In the ovarian cancer context, rhetoric of early detection, intertwined with tropes of unavailability of reliable screening tests, is used to divert attention from larger issues such as the medical community's disregard for women's complaints about disease symptoms. I argue that prioritizing women's symptoms complaints may not necessarily lead to early diagnosis; but it can empower women at a time when their subjective voices are all they can trust given circumstances leading to late diagnosis. Thus, this book challenges popular and medical discourses about ovarian cancer and who is considered at risk, arguing that these discourses, which are neither value- nor cultural-free, silence alternative understandings of the disease. Drawing from current, original data related to ovarian cancer and existing scholarly work on general and specific women's health issues, this book presents a critical feminist and communication studies insight into women's embodied experiences of ovarian cancer and suggests that women's subjective voices matter in uncovering the puzzle about the disease.

Arguments in this book draw from and extend the work of communication, anthropology, critical psychology, and/or feminist scholars such as Emily Martin, Gayle Sulik, Samantha King, Tasha Dubriwny, Kelly Happe, Jane Ussher and colleagues, Michael Hecht (communication theory of identity), Deana Goldsmith (social support), Graham Bodie (dual process theory of supportive message outcomes), Dale Brashers and colleagues (uncertainty management theory), Austin Babrow (problematic integration theory), among others. Emily Martin's (1991, 2001) work on negative framing of the female body and its reproductive functions by the medical community is instructive for my arguments in this book by providing an analysis of cultural and social influences on medical constructions of the female body and the impacts on women's embodiments of their reproductive experiences. Negative depictions of the female reproductive system as a failure, defective, and wasteful hold women accountable for the so-called imperfections of their bodies. Martin's research, in addition to work by Jane Ussher, Janette Perz and Emilee Gilbert on reproductive and sexual health, identity and cancer (e.g., Gilbert et al., 2010a, b, 2011), helps elucidate ovarian cancer survivors' attachments to their bodies and subsequent conceptions of effects of treatments on their sense of self. Similarly, Tasha Dubriwny's (2009, 2010, 2013) work problematizes how dominant media representations of women's health issues depoliticize women's health and support hegemonic constructions of the ideal patient, wife, and mother. In her book *The Vulnerable Empowered Woman: Feminism, Postfeminism, and Women's Health,* Dubriwny (2013) maintains that popular narratives about women's health have created an identity of the "vulnerable empowered woman" who is supposedly empowered through the medical "choices" available to her and thus liable for her own health (Dubriwny, 2013). She argues that such narratives support postfeminist (and neoliberal) tenets of individual responsibility for health and illness. This argument is critical to my analysis of dangers of the blanket promotion of advocacy and self-advocacy in the ovarian cancer context. I stress that narrow focus on behaviors constitutive of self-advocacy and non-self-advocacy essentializes survivors' experiences of self-advocacy and problematically dictates and defines how women should embody their illness experiences. This can engender guilt and shame in survivors who deviate from the supposed norm.

Equally important to my arguments is the work by Kelly Happe on genomics, genetic information and ovarian cancer. In *The Material Gene: Gender, Race, and Heredity after the Human Genome Project* (and other articles), Happe (2013) articulates that genomics (and biomedical discourse and practices broadly) influences and is influenced by cultural perceptions about the body, particularly perceptions about disease, risk, and management of risk. She argues that discourses of genomic medicine (which is supposedly free of political and social influences) explaining disease and the body mainly on the basis of genes and heredity minimize the roles social and environmental categories (e.g., race and gender) play in shaping knowledge about disease and health. Happe (2013) explains controversies in the medical community about oophorectomy's efficacy and how its widespread acceptance supports historical perspectives on the link between reproductive organs and women's health, making oophorectomy an acceptable medical intervention to reduce cancer risk: "When ovariectomy for explicitly cultural reasons fell out of favor, ovarian cancer would present gynecologists with the opportunity to fight a deadly disease requiring nothing less than radical intervention" (p. 71). Knowledge of this historical perspective increases our awareness and encourages us to be curious and wary of medical explanations for radical treatments for ovarian cancer risk and actual disease because "the routinization of oophorectomy for cancer prevention is no less a sociopolitical phenomenon than was routine oophorectomy in the nineteenth century" (Happe, 2013, p. 77). Happe's (2013) focus on "reproductive politics of ovarian cancer genomics research" (p. 18) is particularly significant to the core arguments of this book. She explains that "in ovarian cancer genomics, for example, the intersection of medicine with patriarchy reduces women to reproductive function and desire, a reduction that historically has served to discipline women and force them to adhere to limited, exploitative gender roles" (p. 10). I suggest we keep these issues in mind when examining women's attitudes/demeanor during ovarian cancer treatments and how they find their voices by submitting to grueling treatments (and the medical establishment) as that is the only way they can survive. I contend that ovarian cancer survivors' internalizations of politics around reproductive capabilities of the ovary (as explained by Emily Martin) contribute to shape their embodied experiences of ovarian cancer and communicative responses to effects of treatments. I argue further that the seeming muted communication and knowledge about ovarian cancer derive from prevailing social and medical constructions of the ovary and ovarian cancer, which Happe's work provides context for.

Additionally, Samantha King's classic work on breast cancer and corporate philanthropy provides a critical framework for analyzing advocacy around women's health issues, including ovarian cancer. In her book *Pink Ribbons, Inc.: Breast Cancer and the Politics of Philanthropy,* King (2006) problematizes selective focus on awareness and early detection by professional breast cancer advocacy groups, arguing that this distorts the lived reality of the disease by constructing it as a "unifying issue that is somehow beyond the realms of politics, conflict, or power relations" (p. 112). The successful business strategy by advocacy groups to garner support and funding from political, medical, and corporate actors using nonthreatening and aggressive tactics has diverted attention from core societal issues that contribute to the cancer epidemic. Extending this logic, Gayle Sulik (2011) explains in *Pink Ribbon Blues: How Breast Cancer Culture Undermines Women's Health* that advocacy around breast cancer has created a "pink ribbon culture" where normative beliefs about gender, femininity, women, and the ill are used to raise funds for and market the breast cancer brand. "Most representations of breast cancer use statistics to generate fear and the color pink to evoke innocence and femininity" (p. 137). The pink ribbon culture defines how survivors ought to embody their experiences (i.e., by being optimistic and heroic) and in the process, has produced a normative cancer survivorship discourse that isolates and produces guilt in women who are unable to embody these normative standards. King's and Sulik's arguments illuminate my articulations about ovarian cancer advocacy, self-advocacy, and survivorship.

This book adds to the extant scholarship at the intersection of communication and feminist thinking on politics of the female body and embodiment of women's health issues (e.g., ovarian cancer and breast cancer). It also extends existing work on illness uncertainty management and cancer survivorship by explaining the varied influences on women's experiences of ovarian cancer and conceptions of survivorship, including finances, social support, and treatment aftereffects. Similarly, this book highlights sources (i.e., foci and forms) of uncertainty in the ovarian cancer context and survivors' communicative management of uncertainty. I argue that uncertainty management is integral to ovarian cancer survivorship; it is constantly ongoing and enacted differently by individual women depending on their life circumstances, disease, and contextual factors. Varied enactments of support from relational others are crucial to survivors' experiences of the disease.

OVERVIEW OF CHAPTERS

The ovarian cancer experience begins with a diagnosis, preceded with experience (or nonexperience) of symptoms. In chapter two I discuss events leading to women's diagnosis with ovarian cancer and factors impacting their communicative responses to diagnosis. I term this phase in the ovarian cancer trajectory "(not)making sense" and explain that women's ability to recognize symptoms early or not does not always guarantee early diagnosis because diagnosis requires collaborative efforts among women, physicians, and medical technology. I also discuss issues women take into consideration when disclosing diagnosis to relational others (e.g., relational obligation to disclose health issues and proximity and maturity of children) and the forms of support they receive by disclosing.

I focus on a phase in the ovarian cancer trajectory when survivors are in treatments in chapter three. I name this phase "owning the experience" and analyze the process of making sense of diagnosis and repositioning the self in relation to altering identities and social roles. I discuss active roles women play in defining their experiences and setting boundaries regarding flow of information around their experiences. In the process, women perform expected identities of the ill and women, including acting 'strong,' 'healthy,' and 'normal.' I suggest that this is a strategy by women to forge inner balance and manage their own uncertainties and fears and those of relational others, including spouses, children, parents, and friends. I argue that ovarian cancer survivors simultaneously challenge and reify gender role expectations of the ill and women.

In chapter four, I turn to the period following the end of active treatments to explain the process of ovarian cancer survivorship. Extending the National Coalition for Cancer Survivorship's argument that cancer survivorship begins at diagnosis and continues for the rest of life, I analyze the intentionality of survivorship at the end of active treatments. I do not mean to suggest that survivorship begins at the end of treatment; survivorship is an unending process for some survivors. As indicated by Kylie (65 years old), survivorship is ongoing: "I struggled for three years to become a cancer survivor. My struggle with becoming a cancer survivor was longer and far more intense than fighting cancer." I examine the sources of uncertainty in survivors (e.g., awareness of possible disease recurrence and financial difficulties), how uncertainties were communicatively managed, and the factors that influenced survivors' understandings of their lived experiences.

I extend the discussion of ovarian cancer survivorship in chapter five, where I analyze women's interpretations of physical and psychological consequences of treatments on their sexual self-concept.[2] I focus on the primary female organs associated with ovarian cancer (i.e., ovary and fallopian tubes) and how social perceptions about these organs shape women's communicative responses to effects of treatments on their sexual self-concept. I discuss factors that influence the meaning women construct of their sexual self-concept and highlight how women communicatively manage and negotiate their sexual identities and well-being in the face of a life-threatening disease such as ovarian cancer

In chapter six (which I wrote with Gini Steinke, founder and executive director of Ovarian Cancer Connection [OCC] in Toledo, Ohio) we problematize popular conceptions of self-advocacy in the (ovarian) cancer context and suggest that universal promotion of self-advocacy burdens survivors and encourages individual responsibility for health and illness. To make our argument, we trace history of the women's health movement and (breast) cancer advocacy in Western societies and draw from the work of the OCC to highlight appropriate models of advocacy in the ovarian cancer context. The advocacy we endorse carries promise of encouraging self-advocacy and self-affirmation in the direst circumstances when survivors, due to health reasons, may not be able to embody normative self-advocacy.

The arguments presented in this book aim to delineate how dominant social practices and beliefs support larger medical discourses to impact women's lived experiences of ovarian cancer and therefore, how society comes to understand ovarian cancer. In my analysis, I do not critique women's expressive embodiments of ovarian cancer; my critique centers on hegemonic practices that impact women's lived experiences. I argue for renewed critical examination of discourses around ovarian cancer diagnosis, treatment, survivorship, advocacy and self-advocacy, and a deeper reflection on how these discourses further hegemonic practices that subordinate women and silence their lived experiences.

EXPLANATION OF DATA AND METHOD

Data from which the analysis and arguments in this book are drawn include in-depth interviews[3] and focus groups[4] with ovarian cancer survivors in northwest Ohio and southern Michigan in the United States. At the time data were collected, six of the women were in treatments or about to begin treatments due to recurrences, and one participant was terminal and had stopped treatments. The majority of the women were married and all of them were heterosexual. Eleven of the participants were pre-menopausal at the time of diagnosis and 17 were post-menopausal. The majority of the women described their socioeconomic status as "upper class" or "upper-middle class" and a few described themselves as "struggling" or as "living from paycheck to paycheck." (See table 1.1 for complete demographic information on participants.)

Thirteen women participated in both the interviews and focus groups. In-depth interviews helped understand the subjective experiences of women (Hesse-Biber, 2014), and focus groups placed control over group interactions in the hands of women and allowed for a deeper understanding of the communication codes they used to discuss their experiences (Carey & Smith, 1994; Kitzinger, 1995; Morgan, 1996). These feminist methodologies highlighted survivors' agency through a focus on their definitions of their own experiences and centering their voices in the knowledge co-created (Hesse-Biber, 2014; Jaggar, 2013; Staller & Buch, 2014). The feminist research approach helped give agency to women in this project to name their own experiences and present alternative narratives about the disease, illuminating how each made sense of her experience in her own way. I asked participants questions such as: How have ovarian cancer and its treatments affected your life as a woman, mother, or wife? How have your age, religion, marital status, and socioeconomic status influenced your experience with ovarian cancer? And, what does it mean to be an ovarian cancer survivor? I analyzed women's responses using thematic analysis (Braun & Clark, 2006) guided by a feminist perspective.

In the chapters that follow I trace the lived experience of ovarian cancer through the lenses of women who have lived with and through the disease. But, I acknowledge that women's accounts represented in this book do not tell the entire story about ovarian cancer. My analysis is limited by the homogeneity of women I interviewed, who were mainly married, Caucasian, Christian, and heterosexual. And while I tried to present a comprehensive analysis by drawing from varied scholarly sources, the evidence presented in this book is from the perspectives of survivors alone and not others in their social networks (e.g., children, partners, and caregivers). However, I reviewed relevant literature on how women's partners and social network members reinforce and/or ameliorate the embodied experience of cancer given that the cancer experience is shared (Faulkner, 2016; Goldsmith, 2009). Further, the analysis is shaped by my social position as an African woman with no personal experience of cancer. Practicing reflexivity and my training in feminist research helped minimize my lack of personal experience with cancer. I wrote extensive field notes about my research experiences and constantly reflected on how I could improve the research process and out-

Table 1.1. Demographic Information

Description	Number	% (N=28)
Stage of Disease		
Stage I	6	21.4
Stage II	6	21.4
Stage III	11	39
Stage IV	3	11
Unspecified	2	7
Age[1]		
20–29	2	7
30–39	2	7
40–49	3	11
50–59	10	36
60–69	7	25
70–79	2	7
80–89	2	7
Marital Status		
Married	18	64
Not Married[2]	10	36
Number of Children		
Biological Children	17	60.7
Adopted Children	1	3.6
No Children	10	35.7
Ethnicity		
Caucasian	27	96
Mexican-American	1	4
Level of Education		
High School	5	17.9
Some College/Associate	10	35.7
Bachelors	8	28.6
Some Graduate/Master	5	17.9
Menopausal Status[3]		
Pre-menopausal	11	39
Post-menopausal	17	61
Recurrence Status		
Recurred[4]	8	29
Never Recurred	20	71

1. Age range=23-84; median=58.5.
2. Includes women who were divorced and widowed.
3. Menopausal status at the time of diagnosis.
4. Women whose disease has recurred at least once. Out of this number, three have died.

comes. Through the process, I learned to empathize with women without presuming to *know* their experiences. I disclosed to women that I had not experienced ovarian cancer; a disclosure that gave them some form of control over the data collected, minimized power imbalances between us, and enhanced the intersubjective knowledge produced (Bell, 2014; Staller & Buch, 2014). Giving women the upper hand in the research process helped acknowledge the "epistemic knowledge" they have about their experiences (Collins, 1990). I listened more than I talked; active listening was my way of making women feel comfortable and assuring them that I cared deeply about their experiences. Active, engaged listening can help research participants develop "critical consciousness" about their experiences (Foss & Foss, 1994, p. 42) and can enhance "empathic engagement" in the research process (Atkins, 2015). It is an important gift researchers can give distressed participants (Ellis, 2007). While there are obvious advantages to having authorial knowledge (as opposed to authorial objectivity) on the subject one is researching, including access to the experiences of participants which would have otherwise been missed and ability to ask questions others without personal experience would miss (Segal, 2015), I believe practicing reflexivity and active listening helped address some of the limitations.

NOTES

1. I use "women" and "survivors" interchangeably throughout this book.
2. Sexual health comprises *sexual function* (including desire, arousal/excitement, and orgasm), *sexual self-concept* (including body image, sexual esteem, and sexual self-schema), and *sexual roles and relationships* (including communication and intimacy) (Cleary & Hegarty, 2011; Woods, 1987).
3. The interviews took place face to face in women's homes or coffee shops, over the telephone, or via FaceTime. Each woman received a $20 grocery gift card as compensation. The interviews were semi-structured and lasted between 45 and 120 minutes.
4. A total of four focus groups were conducted; participation ranged from two to four women per group. One group had two participants because some women who agreed to participate in the discussion backed out at the last minute due to health and logistical reasons.

Chapter Two

(Not)making Sense

Receiving an Uncertain Diagnosis

They found a benign ovarian cyst in 2006. [The doctor] followed me every year for five years; I had the CA-125 blood test and transvaginal ultrasound every year. At the time, my breast cancer oncologist thought that the cyst should be removed but my gynecologist explained that so long as it was clear and stable, there was no need to take it out. Then in June 2011, I went in for my annual exam and that cyst had changed dramatically. I was diagnosed with stage 1A ovarian cancer. I was told I did not need chemotherapy because the cancer was in early stages. Then in June 2014 I noticed a lymph node on my leg and I asked my doctor if he thought it was the ovarian cancer returning and he said "no" so we should watch it for a while. Fortunately, two days later I had my six-month appointment with my [breast cancer] oncologist and she was concerned about the lymph nodes. So a biopsy confirmed that I had a recurrence [of ovarian cancer] in two places. I finally found a new [gynecologist], and I wrote to the one whom I had seen for 14 years that I could no longer work with him because I did not trust his judgment anymore concerning my health

Mercy, 58 years, stage[1]

Anger, frustration, and shock describe Mercy's diagnosis with ovarian cancer. As a breast cancer survivor, Mercy had intimate knowledge about her body and health; but she also trusted the opinion of her gynecologist who unfortunately ignored her complaints about ovarian cancer symptoms. She was diagnosed with early stage ovarian cancer when she switched to a different doctor. Mercy's ovarian cancer recurred again and she began treatments shortly after our interview. She was angry with her gynecologist for assuming to know more about his patient and the disease than Mercy herself who embodied the disease. She was right all along about her symptoms but her complaints were ignored and she alone suffered the consequences (not her gynecologist). Mercy is not alone; unfortunately, this is the experience of several ovarian cancer survivors.[2]

Ovarian cancer[3] is the deadliest gynecologic cancer and the fifth leading cause of cancer-related deaths in women in the US (Centers for Disease Control and Prevention; CDC, 2010). More than half of women diagnosed with advanced epithelial ovarian cancer will die within five years (NCI, NIH & US DHHS, 2012). The disease is usually diagnosed at advanced stages (i.e., stages III or IV) because it presents nonspecific symptoms, including swelling and/or pain in the abdomen or pelvis, vaginal bleeding after menopause, constipation, and flatulence (American Cancer Society, 2014; Brain et al., 2014). Thus, the disease has long been described the "silent killer." However, survivors claim the disease presents "shouting" symptoms even at its early stages just that these signs are often attributed to other health conditions because of their generality (Gubar, 2012; Holmes, 2006). Limited knowledge about ovarian cancer, poor prognosis, long, grueling treatments, permanent treatment aftereffects (e.g., neuropathy), and high recurrence and mortality rates contribute to fear and uncertainty about the disease (Cesario et al., 2010; Ferrell et al., 2003; Ozga et al., 2015; Reb, 2007).

In this chapter, I explore the ovarian cancer experience by examining events leading to diagnosis and factors that influence women's interpretations of diagnosis and subsequent disclosure to relational others. In examining women's individual responses to diagnosis, I consider implications disregard for women's subjective knowledge have for their communicative embodiments of the disease. I argue that ovarian cancer is still highly misdiagnosed not only because it presents nonspecific symptoms or because reliable screening tests are nonexistent; but also because women's complaints about symptoms are silenced. There is currently no reliable screening for ovarian cancer[4] as concerns exist about specificity of the United States Food and Drug Administration (FDA)-approved biomarker for the disease, cancer antigen 125 (CA-125). The CA-125 can produce false positive results where elevated antigen levels (as a result of conditions such as "endometriosis, adenomyosis, uterine fibroids, and normal menstruation") are falsely attributed to ovarian cancer (Simmons, Baggerly & Bast, 2013, p. 2). Concerns about the biomarker also relate to how some ovarian cancers do not express CA-125 (Jacobs et al., 1993; Simmons, Baggerly, & Bast, 2013; "NIH develops consensus statement on ovarian cancer," 2004). Recent research exploring potential of human epididymis protein 4 (HE4) to address limitations of CA-125 has found evidence that combining CA-125 and HE4 can be a superior predictor of malignant ovarian cancer than using either CA-125 or HE4 alone (Simmons, Baggerly, & Bast, 2013).

While not underestimating challenges with effective screening tests for ovarian cancer, I argue that these challenges are often highlighted to immobilize women's attempts to be knowledgeable about their bodily processes and to divert attention from failures of the medical community and society to legitimize women's subjective knowledge. Given lack of evidence that early detection of ovarian cancer can reduce disease-related mortality[5] (Cass & Karlan, 2010; Twombly, 2007), I challenge master medical discourses citing lack of reliable screening as a key reason for late diagnosis of ovarian cancer[6] . On the other hand, I maintain that failure to listen to and prioritize women's complaints about symptoms is the core problem the medical community and society have about ovarian cancer. Taking women's complaints seriously should not take second place to finding reliable tests; both should be considered complementary and given equal prominence. Attending to women's complaints about symptoms may not necessarily lead to early diagnosis but can lead to instances where tumors will be detected early, which can consequently impact disease outcomes (Cass & Karlan, 2010). Further, taking women's complaints seriously can be empowering to women and help validate their subjective experiences, especially in instances when their subjective voices and experiences are all they can trust. Constraining women's voices in naming disease symptoms is at the expense of women's lives, and this needs to be challenged. Similarly, I suggest that a critical investigation into women's communicative responses to ovarian cancer diagnosis, including shock and anger, can point to multiple targets for these emotive expressions (e.g., the disease and the medical establishment), and challenge conventional beliefs that these are typical responses to a cancer diagnosis.

I name the diagnostic phase in the ovarian cancer trajectory "(not)making sense" because diagnosis and circumstances surrounding it do not make sense to women. Any cancer diagnosis does not make sense (Faulkner, 2016). But ovarian cancer diagnosis is complicated because the disease presents nonspecific symptoms (e.g., nausea, diarrhea or constipation, pelvic or abdominal pains, and bloating; Rossing, Wicklund, Cushing-Haugen & Weiss, 2010), which, to a larger extent, neither women nor physicians are able to accurately interpret. The small percentage of women who recognize symptoms and complain about them are not taken seriously. This is counterintuitive to rhetoric asking women to be proactive about their health and to know their bodies, given that cooperation among women, physicians, and medical tests (e.g., ultrasounds) is needed to diagnose ovarian cancer. The (not)making sense phase describes the period between onset of symptoms and start of treatments for ovarian cancer. It is a period of intense uncertainty. The period can span weeks or months during which women live on the borderlines of health and illness, hope and hopelessness, voice and voiceless as they silently question if changes in their bodies point to disease. Knowing they are voicing speeches of their bodies but these are not authenticated by external bodies, including physicians and the medical establishment, can be frustrating, protract diagnosis, and hinder women's proactive involvement in their health. Women are forced into silence—a silence some attempt to break by consulting multiple doctors (and the added cost and stress that brings). Many women receive late diagnosis, indicating that try as they may to prove otherwise, control over their health is not entirely in their hands. However, each woman's situation is different, meaning that the process of diagnosis is experienced differently. Here, I examine factors that underlie these differences in experience.

NOT/RECOGNIZING SYMPTOMS

The diagnostic phase in the ovarian cancer trajectory begins with the experience of nonspecific symptoms such as bloating, flatulence, lack of appetite, spotting between menses, back and lower abdominal pain. Many women and their physicians, most of the time, are unable to connect these symptoms to ovarian cancer because of their vagueness and because of factors such as women's age, overall health status, and family history of cancer. Women who experience ovarian cancer symptoms naturally get worried and casually complain to people in their social networks, but do not anticipate symptoms pointing to a serious disease. Because ovarian cancer is not in their forecasts or in their daily vocabulary as a result of how disease risk factors are promoted (I discuss this below), women tone down communication about symptoms. They complain only when symptoms and pains become persistent, or talk about symptoms as a side-conversation (i.e., they talk about symptoms casually). Talking about symptoms casually prompts a casual response. For instance, Grace (26 years, stage I) stated, "I kept noticing that my stomach was getting bigger and I would tell my friends how I was losing weight but my stomach was protruding and it was rock hard. And my friends would say 'no, you are fine; it is just your stomach.' I was like something is wrong but no one believed me." Aside from her age which made friends oblivious that her symptoms could be ovarian cancer, Grace's communication about her symptoms set the tone for how her friends responded. She discussed her symptoms in the context of weight loss because she lacked knowledge about ovarian cancer and did not consider herself at risk. I argue that perceptions about age and risk factors for ovarian cancer intersect with other factors (e.g., communication and knowledge about disease) to impact reaction to disease symptoms.

On the surface, it seems justified to assume that women communicate disease symptoms non-assertively, conforming to the supposed natural disposition of all women. However, it is important to realize that women lack the necessary vocabulary to express what they experience in their bodies. Martha Holmes (2006) accurately observes that "ovarian tumors . . . are not part of our daily vocabulary" (p. 491)—a view echoed in a 2008 study by

Bankhead and colleagues who found that ovarian cancer survivors experienced disease symptoms for about 12 months prior to diagnosis, but "the terminology used by women to name their symptoms did not always accurately describe the symptoms they experienced" (p. 1012). This points to limited public knowledge about ovarian cancer (Carter, DiFeo, Bogie, Zhang, & Sun, 2014; National Ovarian Cancer Coalition, n.d.).

Popular and scientific literature identify ovarian cancer risk factors to include family history of ovarian and/or breast cancer (for epithelial ovarian cancer), some gene mutations (i.e., BRCA 1/2), delayed childbearing, late menopause, early menstruation, and some environmental factors (Fleming, Beaugié, Haviv, Chenevix-Trench & Tan, 2006; Lalwani, Shanbhogue, Vikram, Nagar, Jagirdar and Prasad, 2010). By this categorization, young women, women who are healthy and active, and those with no family history of cancer are generally not considered at risk of the disease. Thus, the disease is not on the radar of many women and physicians. Ovarian cancer is not the first disease gynecologists/physicians think about when women complain about symptoms because, among other things, physicians are trained to believe the disease does not present symptoms at early stages (Twombly, 2007). This view about the disease continues to be perpetuated despite survivors' repeated assertions that the disease presents symptoms even at early stages[7] (Ferrell et al., 2003; Gubar, 2012; Twombly, 2007). To clarify some of these misconceptions about ovarian cancer symptoms and to help with early detection, three cancer groups, including the American Cancer Society, the Society of Gynecologic Oncologists, and the Gynecologic Cancer Foundation, released a consensus statement in June 2007 arguing for recognition of common symptoms of the disease—what they termed "ovarian cancer symptom index" (Twombly, 2007). The symptom index was developed based on experiences of ovarian cancer survivors (Twombly, 2007). Despite doubts about the predictive value of a symptom index, scholars have suggested that the index may be more effective at early detection of the disease than any screening test (Cass & Karlan, 2010). A study using the symptom index found that ovarian cancer presented symptoms at early and late stages and that symptoms were 10 times more likely to present in women susceptible to the disease than in the general population (Rossing, Wicklund, Cushing-Haugen & Weiss, 2010).

The strength of these research studies gives credence to the need to validate women's voices and personal health experiences, and calls for a reconfiguration of ovarian cancer risk factors, criteria for determining who may or may not be at risk, and steps taken to manage risk. These issues are intertwined and influence the type of medical advice and treatments women receive and how women embody their experiences. According to Kelly Happe (2013) "Developments in ovarian cancer detection and treatment—such as more and more calls for genetic testing and strongly worded recommendations for aggressive, sometimes experimental, procedures—suggest that in the practice of ovarian cancer research and treatment, heredity itself is disease" (p. 82). Myopic focus on mutated genes for determining disease risk (and treatments) obscures attention to other possible causes of ovarian cancer (e.g., environmental factors), seeks to blame BRCA carriers for getting cancer, emphasizes individual responsibility for health, and limits women's reproductive autonomy (Happe, 2006). BRCA/genetic testing is accorded high status in the medical community not only because of its ability to screen but also its potential to supposedly protect at-risk women and prevent disease (through prophylactic surgery; Happe, 2013). Prevention in this sense means "surveillance not of the individual but of likely occurrences of disease, anomalies, deviant behavior to be minimized and healthy behavior maximized" (Rainbow, 1992, p. 242). A large consensus among the research and medical community is for BRCA-positive women to consider oophorectomy (i.e., surgical removal of ovaries; Happe, 2006). (Although some organizations like the US National Human Genome Research Institute do not explicitly endorse oophorectomy because of concerns about the procedure leading to other cancers later on; Happe, 2013). With increasing evidence of locating cancerous cells during oophorectomy, the procedure is justified on grounds of its ability to lead to early detection of ovarian cancer. In emphasizing oophorectomy, the medical community privileges the ovary's reproductive functions over other roles it performs in the body "by making motherhood the only acceptable reason for postponing oophorectomy" (Happe, 2013, p. 94).

Further, promoting genetic testing to determine cancer risk serves the commercial interests of medical and pharmaceutical corporations which stand to benefit from increased recommendation of genetic testing for cancer risk management (Happe, 2006). Commercialization of genetic testing has given a new meaning to risk, conceptualized as women with a BRCA mutation (not just those with family history of cancer). Preventative treatment (e.g., oophorectomy) is recommended for these new "risk subjects" by age 35 or after childbearing is completed (Happe, 2006, p. 177). This recommendation is framed in the language of empowerment, choice, and control; but what is not highlighted is the fear, uncertainties, and constraints "choice" and "control" put on women's reproductive autonomy. What is not highlighted is the "constrained field of risk" within which women with BRCA1/2 mutations must exercise their supposed reproductive choices (Happe, 2017, p. 352). At-risk women who fail to remove their ovaries and fallopian tubes after age 35 are considered culpable for neglecting cancer risk at their own risk (Happe, 2017)—a notion that disciplines the female body and promotes individual responsibility for health and disease.

Ironically, genetic tests do not detect disease/tumor; they detect risk, which is now managed/treated as actual disease. Because risk is abstract and cannot be manipulated, what is "manipulated is a woman's body, in this case her reproductive organs [i.e., ovaries and fallopian tubes]" (Happe, 2006, p. 181). Happe (2006) argues that women "embody heredity" (p. 173) in that rhetoric of ovarian cancer risk impacts how women (and relational others) experience risk and steps they take to manage risk, including removal of healthy ovaries. Indeed many at-risk women consider removal of the ovaries a means to regain control over their bodies and health albeit with some risks, including compromising relational and sexual self-identities (Hallowell & Lawton, 2002). Popularity of the genetic risk rhetoric affects family members of ovarian cancer survivors who may feel compelled to get genetic testing to determine their susceptibility (Happe, 2006) and an additional burden (and responsibility of guilt) to disclose positive test results (Hallowell et al., 2006)

This is part of the problem with blanket promotion of "choice" and "risk" in women's health care critical culture and feminist scholars seek to draw attention to. These scholars argue that master discourses of choice and risk ignore inequalities in how the concepts are structured and applied (Dubriwny, 2013; Fixmer-Oraiz, 2014; Happe, 2013; Hayden, 2009; Lippman, 1999; Silva, 2011) and promote postfeminist tenets of an empowered, independent woman who is free to make her own choices (Kissling, 2013). They note that medical explanations of ovarian cancer risk work to surveil and control women's bodies by sanctioning when and who can exercise her reproductive autonomy (Happe, 2006). Extending this argument, this book suggests that the rhetoric of "risk" in the context of ovarian cancer serves to limit access to and knowledge about their bodies and health for women classified not at-risk while increasing uncertainty and fear in those marked as at-risk. Categorizing some women as at higher risk of the disease than others leaves those supposedly not at-risk in the dark in terms of knowledge about the disease, and contributes to efforts to take away women's rights to understand their bodies and health and place it in the hands of the medical establishment (Ussher, 1989). Also disquieting is that not all women considered at-risk of hereditary breast and ovarian cancer are eligible for predictive testing (Hallowell, 2006); yet genetic testing is promoted as the solution to early detection of ovarian cancer (Happe, 2013).

RECEIVING LATE/MISDIAGNOSIS

Inability to accurately interpret disease symptoms may lead women to use physical activity and other means (e.g., eating gluten-free and diary-free foods) to manage symptoms, or watch symptoms for improvements. Some women may follow their intuition or advice from relational ones and visit the hospital, where after several tests are run they are diagnosed and treated for conditions such as pre-menopausal symptoms, urinary tract infections, indigestion, or back/hip pains. Others are told their symptoms do not exist (i.e., symptoms "are in your head") and are sent home. When symptoms do not get better, women return to the hospital and persist until they receive a (late) diagnosis of ovarian cancer. Unlike some cancers (e.g., breast cancer) which can be diagnosed through self-examination, ovarian cancer cannot be self-diagnosed. Ovarian cancer is detected with the assistance of medical technology because the associated organs—the ovaries and fallopian tubes—are not readily accessible to women because of their location in the female body (Holmes, 2006). In this case, the extent to which women are able to exercise "control" and "choice" over their health is limited by lack of technical and/or medical know-how and access to all body parts. This can be frustrating especially as women's "gut feelings" about something being wrong in their bodies are not scientific hence considered not credible. Lacking direct access to all parts of their bodies limits the agency women exercise over their bodies and how they interpret and communicate knowledge about their health.

Mediated knowledge of and access to women's bodies is further demonstrated in how surgical procedures are used to confirm suspicions of cancer from ultrasound, pelvic examinations, and/or blood tests (i.e., CA-125 or HE4) and to stage the disease. Ovarian cancer is diagnosed and staged surgically (Prat, 2014). Thus, most women go into surgery without knowing for sure that they have ovarian cancer—a situation that exacerbates uncertainty and distress upon final diagnosis. The uncertainty women experience between the onset of symptoms and diagnosis is undeniable (Ferrell et al., 2003; Ozga et al., 2015; Reb, 2007). Women hope and pray their symptoms are not cancer or that if anything at all the disease will be in its early stages. Depending on the outcome of surgery, women must adjust hope and find ways to embrace reality. Women have to completely switch their mindsets from hoping their symptoms will not be cancer to modifying their roles and identities, which can be difficult to communicate about (Miller, 2015).

It can be a matter of days or weeks when scans show tumors and when women have surgery and start treatments (mostly chemotherapy or radiation). The rapid progression of events helps explain why women are "shocked," "numbed," "frozen," "stunned," and "surprised" upon diagnosis, for good or bad reasons. Expecting symptoms not to be cancer but they end up being cancer, or expecting to be diagnosed with advanced disease and instead get diagnosed with early stage disease, or expecting to be diagnosed early stage and it turns out to be late stage all can evoke shock, numbness, or surprise. These reactions are fueled by women's age, health status at the time of diagnosis, and family history of cancer. For instance, Lyne (60 years, stage II) explained, "When I got news of my diagnosis, I was like, "okay, what do you mean by ovarian cancer? We do not have ovarian cancer in my family." Esther (48 years, stage III) also mentioned that "I certainly would not have considered myself a likely candidate for ovarian cancer because I had no family history of breast or ovarian cancer. I ate very healthy within my ideal body weight; I ran a few days a week. I was overall in good health; I had no health issues going on. It was a very big surprise, the diagnosis." These reasons contribute to make the diagnosis disquieting for women.

Shock at diagnosis can also emanate from receiving a clean bill of health weeks earlier only to be diagnosed with cancer later. Women cannot correlate symptoms they are experiencing with ovarian cancer because they do not expect to be declared healthy and at the same time have ovarian cancer developing in their bodies. For instance, Juliet (59 years, stage II) noted, "I went to my gynecologist in August for my annual exam and everything came back fine and six weeks later, I was in surgery [for ovarian cancer]. That was how fast it all happened. It was never explained to me that the annual pap smear does not detect ovarian cancer; and the symptoms of the disease were also not explained to me so when I was having the symptoms, I did not know what they were." As stated previously, an implicit target of women's shock and anger is the medical establishment which has confused women and the public with contradictory information about the disease and its risk factors. Ovarian cancer is framed as a medical mystery only the medical community can understand. And, a great number of women erroneously think Papanicolaou (Pap) test screens for ovarian cancer.

Pap test is the only recommended population-based routine screening for a gynecologic cancer (i.e., cervical cancer) in the United States and while knowledge and awareness about the test is high among the general public, there are also misconceptions about its ability to screen for other cancers, including ovarian cancer. A study conducted by Hawkins and colleagues (2011) to assess the *Inside Knowledge: Get the Facts about Gynecologic Cancer* campaign[8] found that over 80 percent of women accurately acknowledged that Pap test screened for cervical cancer. However, the majority of the participants also believed the test screened for other diseases, including ovarian cancer (about 40 percent of participants believed Pap test screened for ovarian cancer). Cooper, Polonec and Gelb (2010) also observed similar findings in their study where "A few participants remarked that regular Pap testing was especially vital to detect ovarian cancer" (p. 521). Hawkins and colleagues (2011) concluded that "Misconceptions about the purpose of the Pap test in routine screening could have deleterious effects among women who may mistakenly believe that a normal Pap test result indicates the absence of disease or problems in areas that were never addressed by the test" (p. 514). This was the experience of Juliet (explained above) and many ovarian cancer survivors.

Everything women know and have been practicing health and wellness-wise does not seem to hold true anymore after an ovarian cancer diagnosis. Most women do all the "right things," including eating healthy, exercising, and having annual gynecological exams, yet get diagnosed with ovarian cancer. A diagnosis, thus, not only shakes the core of their belief systems; it also affects their symbols and patterns of communication. Being healthy and active, having no history of cancer in the family and at the same time being diagnosed with cancer means that women need a new set of communication symbols to express their circumstances in ways that make sense to themselves first based on their new roles and identities, then to others in their social networks. The old framework for interpreting health and wellness cannot adequately explain women's new experiences; their physical states of health contrast their understandings of risk factors of cancer. This book suggests that uncertainties about health women experience upon diagnosis are partly due to the fact that they can no longer trust anything and anybody—their bodies, the medical establishment, and belief systems. Yet, they need to keep hope alive.

Women communicate their shock, anger, frustration, and disappointment variedly. Some cry while others do not. For some women, crying is an expression of vindication that they are right about their symptoms. For others, crying provides closure to the frustrations of not being listened to—a closure that marks the beginning of a fight for life. For instance, Rose (55 years, stage III) mentioned, "when [the doctor] told me I had cancer, I did not cry because I had cancer, I cried because I was right and I knew something was wrong." Rose felt relieved and vindicated; finally, the speech of her body was validated resulting in a diagnosis, although belatedly. Similarly, Gena (79 years, stage III) stated, "I saw about 11 different doctors who kept giving me anti-depressants because they were treating me as depressed hysterical woman. When I got the diagnosis, I was like 'I am not crazy; I know there was something wrong.' When you do not feel good for so long and nobody can find anything and suddenly they find something, you are like 'hey, I am not crazy.'" I argue that listening to women and considering them partners in their own health can help address some of the emotional stresses women experience upon diagnosis. This may or may not help with early detection, but it can help women feel valued and empowered knowing that their subjective experiences are respected. Statistics, backed by the lived realities of women, are telling but will the medical and academic research communities listen?

COMMUNICATING DIAGNOSIS

Communicating an ovarian cancer diagnosis can be a difficult undertaking. This is partly due to the risks associated with revealing private information (e.g., loss of control; Petronio & Durham, 2015) and because women themselves may just be beginning to comprehend the diagnosis. Thus, women exercise great care, judgment, and control over how and to whom they disclose their diagnosis (Donovan-Kicken, Tollison & Goins, 2011). To maintain relational stability and to protect themselves and relational others who did not witness the diagnosis (Caughlin & Vangelisti, 2009; Donovan-Kicken & Caughlin, 2010; Goldsmith, Miller, & Caughlin, 2008), women carefully calculate the timing of the disclosure. Some choose to wait until after surgery to inform loved ones while others relay the news as soon as tumors are suspected and/or found[9] . The styles women use depend on the maturity of their children, proximity to loved ones, family communication pattern, and other family and/or health issues going on at the time of the diagnosis (e.g., death in the family or health problems with other family members). Family members who are too young to understand or those who have other health problems that may inhibit their ability to comprehend and help women process the diagnosis may be spared the news or have the news broken down for them. For example, Andrea (43 years, stage III) described her cancer as "peas" for her nine-year-old son to understand.

Women disclose out of relational obligation and a need to receive social support. In (familial) relationships, there is an unstated obligation to share health information for one's sake and also for the sake of other family members (Donovan-Kicken, Tollison & Goins, 2012; Greenberg & Smith, 2016). Women, thus, disclose the diagnosis first to those in their immediate families; some later use social media and other avenues to inform others about the diagnosis. For example, Stella's (63 years, stage II) children were aware of her health condition so she felt they needed to know when she received the cancer diagnosis. She said, "[My children] knew I was seeing a physician for my hip pain but I knew I had to call them and tell them when [the doctors] found the tumor. I did not call them right away; I waited until I had the CT scan [results]. I asked them to call me when they were able to talk and not driving and they all called me eventually." Stella considered it part of her obligations as a mother to disclose her diagnosis to her children; but also important to her was the well-being of her children, hence the timing and manner in which she disclosed the news. She was deliberate about her disclosure and asked her children to call her without giving them any hint about what they would discuss. She made sure they were in safe environments (i.e., not driving) to receive the news. Stella also considered it her duty to make sure her children had accurate information to act on so she waited until the diagnosis was confirmed. Stella felt she did not immediately need the support of her grown children because they lived far away and because her husband was with her to provide immediate assistance. Thus, available support and proximity are factors that may influence how and when an ovarian cancer diagnosis is disclosed to relational others.

The obligation to disclose diagnosis can be distressing if women have young children at home. Women worry that young children are incompetent to understand a cancer diagnosis and that exposing children to news about cancer undermines their responsibility to protect their children. Yet, they also feel it is their job to be open to their children to the best of their abilities. This relational role tension adds to the emotional work involved in disclosing an ovarian cancer diagnosis. For instance, Esther (48 years, stage III) remarked, "I would say telling [my children] when I was first diagnosed was awful; everybody cried. And when a child hears 'cancer' they automatically think 'are you going to die?'" Children can be blunt in their communication, which can contradict women's resolve to fight cancer and add to an already emotionally-charged diagnosis. Thus, women's choice of style and language to communicate a cancer diagnosis is influenced by a desire to claim control over the situation and to calm the fears of relational others. In communicating their diagnosis, women consider the risks not only to themselves but also to their loved ones (Charmaz, 1991).

To allay the fears of young children, women tone down their diagnosis by using non-threatening language to communicate it. They use language their children can relate to. Consider how Andrea (43 years, stage III) disclosed her diagnosis to her youngest child. She explained, "When we got home [from the hospital], we did not want to call it "cancer" in front of my smallest child who was 9 years old. We told him that I just had some infections in my stomach and I am going to have surgery and it is going to make mom's hair fall off. We did not call it 'cancer' so we thought of something that I really do not like and I hate peas so we called it 'peas.' Mom has peas." Andrea configured the language that worked best for her child. Communicating a cancer diagnosis to young children adds to the complexities women must navigate as they try to make sense of their diagnosis, and presents an ovarian cancer diagnosis as involving multiple communicative processes and tensions beyond receiving the diagnosis from physicians.

A desire to protect loved ones when disclosing an ovarian cancer diagnosis also means that when women perceive that disclosing will do more harm than good, they choose not to disclose. Women's sense of inner strength is tied to the well-being of their loved ones such that disclosure is for their own good as well as for their loved ones—everyone in their social network need to be on the same page. Thus, Rose (55 years, stage III) did not tell her mother, who had Alzheimer's disease, about her diagnosis because she was not in a position to understand. Similarly, Ann (65 years) did not disclose her diagnosis to her mother who had Lewy body disease and was grieving the death of her son (Ann's brother). Ann explained she did not see the point in burdening her mother with her diagnosis seeing that she was emotionally distraught at the time. Here, we see an intermingling of women's roles/identities as cancer survivors and caregivers and how negotiating these roles influence their meaning making processes. In the process some women's cancer experiences take backstage as they simultaneously manage the health situations of other family members (Dorgan et al., 2014). For instance, Ann explained she did not give much thought to her ovarian cancer diagnosis and treatment because she was diagnosed at an early stage and did not have chemotherapy or radiation treatment (she had surgery); but also because a lot of health issues happened in her family around the time of her diagnosis. She said, "I don't think about [my diagnosis]. I had the cancer and six months later my mother passed away and six months after that a close friend of mine got pancreatic cancer and I did four trips back and forth to Utah [to visit my friend]. My friend died in 3 months."

Receiving Support through Disclosure

Disclosing a diagnosis can present opportunities for women to receive support from relational others. However, it can also pose risks such as loss of privacy, autonomy, and support (Charmaz, 1991; Faulkner, 2016). As I explain in chapter 3, some friends deserted women upon learning about their cancer diagnosis. On the whole, social support is crucial to the cancer experience. Social support in the context of health includes the structure of one's social networks and the functions these perform for him/her (Schaefer et al., 1981; Semmer et al., 2008; Uchino, 2004; Umberson, Crosnoe & Reczek, 2010). Women's emotions are raw when they are given a cancer diagnosis thus they need all the support they can count on. Support women receive by disclosing diagnosis can be significant in helping put the diagnosis into perspective. Women mainly receive emotional[10] and tangible[11] support from relational others. Some close friends and/or family members may move in to stay with women to help with caregiving, including providing transportation and food during treatment. For example, Patricia stated, "My middle daughter moved in with me when I had my treatments to watch me and help cook and check on me to make sure I was okay." Marie (54 years, stage I) also said when her sister heard about her diagnosis "she got on a flight right away to come stay with us for two weeks."

Because of the potential face threats tangible support can pose (Floyd & Ray, 2016) some women choose to refuse this type of support. Rose (55 years, stage III) explained that people had offered to help her during treatments but she decided not to accept it. She said, "people would say, 'oh, if you need a ride let me know' but you just don't want to ask. I would drive myself [to treatments] even though I would stop every 10–15 minutes to throw up; I just don't ask for help." Rose explained how a routine activity such as "taking a shower that normally should take 20 minutes turned into a couple of hours' ordeal" but she would still not ask for help. Mercy (58 years, stage I) also said she chose to go through treatments alone. She stated, "I went by myself. I wanted it that way. I wanted to go in, have chemotherapy and come home and rest; I didn't want to feel like I have to entertain anybody or worry about them. I just wanted to go in and get it done."

Some support women receive involves more than doing something *for* them to include *being* with them. This is when relational others provide support by being there as women's "calming factor." Sometimes support is most effective when it involves *being present* rather than *doing something*. For example, Andrea's family members shaved their heads to show solidarity during her chemotherapy; an act that was helpful to her coming to terms with losing her hair. This gesture, among others, highlights the effectiveness of providing emotional support through nonverbal immediacy behavior (Jones, 2004). Some women appreciate support provided through nonverbal immediacy because it speaks to them right where they are at.

The dual process theory of supportive message outcomes (Bodie & Burleson, 2008; Bodie & MacGeorge, 2015) suggests outcomes of supportive messages depend on motivation and ability of recipients to evaluate message content. The theory posits further that qualities of recipients and the situation (i.e., severity of the situation and intensity of emotional distress) can impact motivation and ability to elaborate on supportive message. For instance, emotionally distressing situations can increase one's motivation and need for supportive messages; however, intensity of the distress can hinder the recipient's ability to process messages (Bodie, 2012; Bodie & Burleson, 2008; Bodie & MacGeorge, 2015). Highly stressful situations (e.g., a devastating diagnosis or a stressful public speaking event) can decrease motivation and ability to process supportive messages. In such instances, environmental cues, including nonverbal immediacy (i.e., simply being present), can influence appraisal of the supportive message (Bodie, 2012; Bodie & Burleson, 2008; Bodie & MacGeorge, 2015). Because relational others may not have experienced cancer themselves, telling women everything will be okay (i.e., providing support using high verbal content) may not be effective because relational others do not know that for sure. This is pertinent given circumstances surrounding women's diagnosis that destabilized their belief systems and fueled distrust for the medical establishment. But what relational others know and can do is be in the moment with women, walking side-by-side with them. Communicating support through high nonverbal immediacy is considered effective in established interpersonal relationships as it communicates interpersonal warmth, closeness and availability (Jones, 2004).

RACING AGAINST TIME

Once diagnosis is confirmed, women work on treatment plans with their team of physicians and begin treatments almost immediately. Women jump into action and go aggressively after the disease. This is the best response they can give given that diagnosis is made late and further delay can be lethal and because ovarian cancer is aggressive and deadly. Women, thus, lack time to process their diagnosis. This explains why many of them need time to process what has happened when treatments (i.e., chemotherapy or radiation) are underway and they are sure they have the disease under control. For instance, Andrea noted, "It happened so fast; it came and went before I even knew it. I do not even know if I have had time to process everything. Because you are given that diagnosis and you are like, 'okay, let us act now; let us do it.' So you do it and you just keep going and you do not give yourself the time to think about it." Women are in a race against time to save their lives. Women feel control over their health is somewhat back in their hands and they make sure to exercise it to the fullest. It is a different thing not knowing what is going on in your body; it is a different thing knowing something is wrong but not having others to agree with you on what you know is wrong; and it is a different thing having the speech of your body corroborated through an uncertain diagnosis. Women are in charge once again; they can move as fast as they desire. They can push their bodies to the limit and undergo as many treatments as possible; but the effectiveness of these actions is contingent on a host of factors, medical and otherwise, outside the control of women. Ovarian cancer is not handled alone; it takes collaborative efforts; hence, there is a problem when everyone/thing involved is not moving at the same wavelength. This makes the "fight" and "control" rhetoric problematic in the ovarian cancer context because it ignores the failures and inadequacies of other parties involved, including physicians and health insurance programs/policies. Women simply cannot "fight" alone.

It is also important to underscore that having limited time to process diagnosis is not distressing to some women as it gives them the opportunity to channel their energy into treatments and into determining to survive. They have no time for negative energy and to ruminate over their prognosis; no time for "pity-party." For instance, Christie (59 years, stage III) stated, "It was really quick from when I had my diagnosis and had to go into surgery; it was very quick and I did not have much time to think about it, which is not a bad thing because when you got time to think about it, it is very scary." It is very scary particularly when women's chances of survival are not definite as treatments can go either way or when they are told point-blank that the prognosis is poor. Chelsea (56 years, stage III) was told her prognosis was not good and that she should "put her affairs in order." She said, "I was thinking I am going to die within a few weeks. I sat in my home crying as I met with the funeral director; it was traumatic. First, you just received the diagnosis that you have cancer, then you hear that you needed to get your final affairs in order, and it is not that I have a husband or a mother living that was going to take care of my final affairs. That sent me into a state of shock." Putting final or temporary affairs (i.e., situations with work, family, and finances) in order takes time and a toll on women. Women who lack support in terms of immediate family or relational partners are faced with the challenge of managing these issues alone at the same time as they process their diagnosis and plan a treatment course. These factors highlight how the shock women experience at diagnosis pertains not only to the diagnosis itself but also to the task of processing potential death and lack of social buffer.

Women with strong social and financial buffers process the shock of diagnosis differently than those who lack these resources. Those in the latter category face a double burden at diagnosis (i.e., processing diagnosis and putting social and financial affairs in order) which can have rippling effects for the reminder of their cancer journey. Women's social and financial circumstances provide important lenses to understand the ovarian cancer experience and survivorship process (see chapter 4). It is important to consider the intersectional effects of these issues in addition to stage of disease and treatment regimen to better understand the ovarian cancer experience.

The process of (not)making sense of an ovarian cancer diagnosis is explained in figure 2.1.

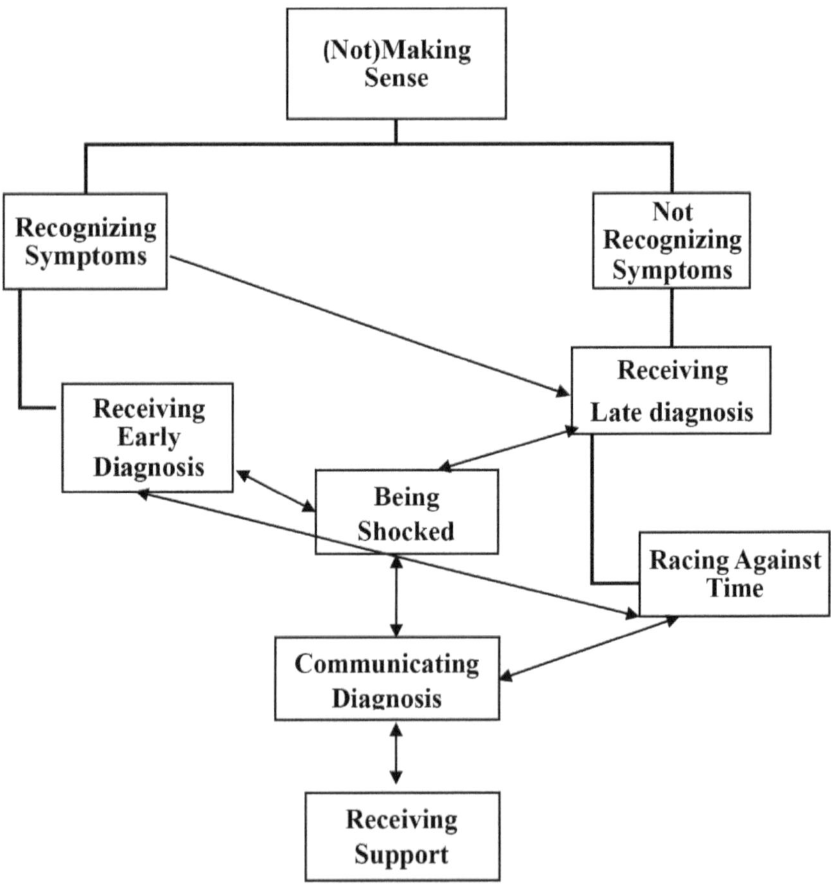

Figure 2.1. The Process of (Not)Making Sense of an Ovarian Cancer Diagnosis

Listening to women's complaints about disease symptoms may not lead to early diagnosis or reduce mortality. However, it can affect disease outcome by reducing "tumor burden at diagnosis" (Cass & Karlan, 2010). Importantly, it can legitimize women's subjective experiences and empower them to fight the disease how they choose to. There is still a lot that is unknown about ovarian cancer; thus, it is important that the voices of women who have lived with and through the disease are considered critical to unlocking the puzzle about the disease. Circumstances surrounding ovarian cancer (diagnosis), including undermining of women's complaints and excuses about lack of reliable screening tests, work to disadvantage women and the advancement of knowledge about women's health, and have implications for experience of the disease. How do these challenges manifest in women's embodiment of the disease in the reminder of the illness trajectory? Do the mindsets and attitudes with which women go through treatments reflect their experiences with the medical establishment, physicians, and belief systems during the diagnostic phase? Do these experiences and beliefs about the disease coerce women into submission during treatment? How do women challenge/oppose systemic efforts to silence them with grueling treatments? What communicative strategies do women use to determine their own lived experiences once when feel a sense of control over their health? I address these questions in the next chapter.

NOTES

1. I include survivors' age and stage of disease to provide context and help readers understand how each woman's unique circumstance contribute to her experience of ovarian cancer.
2. I adopt the National Coalition for Cancer Survivorship's (NCCS) definition of a cancer survivor. NCCS defines survivorship as "from the time of diagnosis and for the balance of life" (http://www.canceradvocacy.org/about-us/our-mission/).
3. Ovarian cancer is not a single disease; it is a general term used to describe cancers that originate in the ovary (Committee on the State of the Science in Ovarian Cancer Research et al., 2016).
4. Kelly Happe (2013) suggests the rhetoric of lack of reliable screening for ovarian cancer is linked to the elevated status and commercialization of BRCA tests as these are considered able to both screen and protect at-risk women (see pp. 80-81).
5. Prognosis of ovarian cancer depends on a host of factors, including early diagnosis, cancer cell type (i.e., high-grade serous, mucinous, endometrioid, clear cell, or low-grade serous), and whether the tumor is benign, malignant, and intermediate (borderline tumor). Some tumors (e.g., low-grade serous carcinoma, mucinous carcinoma, endometrioid carcinoma, malignant Brenner tumor, and clear cell carcinoma) grow slowly while others (e.g., high-grade serous carcinoma) "evolve rapidly, metastasize early in their course, and are highly aggressive" (Shih & Kurman, 2004, p. 1513).
6. In the case of breast cancer, Samantha King (2006) argues that potential of mammogram for early detection of the disease does "not necessarily improve the survival of patients, but rather extend the amount of time in which women bear knowledge of their condition" (p. 38).
7. The important roles ovarian cancer survivors play in changing perspectives about the disease is discussed in chapter 6.

8. The *Inside Knowledge: Get the Facts about Gynecologic Cancer* campaign was instituted by the Centers for Disease Control and Prevention (CDC) in collaboration with the U.S. Department of Health and Human Services' Office on Women's Health in support of the Gynecologic Cancer Education and Awareness Act of 2005, or Johanna's Law (signed into law in 2007 to raise awareness about cervical, ovarian, uterine, vaginal, and vulvar cancers) (Hawkins et al., 2011; Cooper, Polonec & Gelb, 2010).

9. Some women do not personally disclose diagnosis to others depending on the severity of their conditions and who was with them when they were diagnosed.

10. Emotional support is the "communication behavior enacted by one party with the intent of helping another cope effectively with emotional distress" (Burleson, 2010, p. 179).

11. Tangible support includes providing direct/material aid or services for people in need (Cohen & McKay, 1984; Uchino, 2004).

Chapter Three

Setting Boundaries and Distancing Selves

Owning the Lived Experience of Ovarian Cancer

> *When I was first diagnosed I sent a letter to my [work] colleagues letting them know that I would answer any question about ovarian cancer they needed to know; I just do not want questions about prognosis because I do not know what my prognosis was. So I set those boundaries and I think that was helpful to people because I let them know right away what I was most comfortable talking about and what I was not.*
>
> *Esther, 48 years, stage III*

The above quotation exemplifies the quagmire many (ovarian) cancer survivors face in a desire to determine their own experiences while concomitantly connecting with others. Esther is a registered nurse living with recurrent ovarian cancer. She was diagnosed when she was in the middle of finishing her master's degree. She did not consider herself at risk of ovarian cancer, because there was no history of cancer in her family, she lived a healthy lifestyle, and was in good health overall. Esther explained she had no problem sharing her experience with others to educate about the disease; but also noted it was important for her to set the parameters within which the discussions took place. She set boundaries around her experience in order to foster meaningful conversation about the disease, protect her sense of control over the disease, and control what and who could influence her lived experience of the disease.

The ovarian cancer experience is wrought with uncertainties partly because of unpredictable disease progression and high recurrence and mortality rates (Fitch, Gray & Franssen, 2001; Hipkins, Whitworth, Tarrier & Jayson,

2004; Lockwood-Rayermann, 2006) and because of circumstances leading to diagnosis. Coupled with this, physical and psychological effects of treatments present identity and social role challenges for women. Thus, it is significant that some survivors are upfront about their feelings, take steps to protect their sense of self, and actively manage contradictory behaviors and messages. As survivors have yet to fully comprehend the unexpected and sometimes sudden changes diagnosis and treatments made to their identities and social roles, opportunities may arise during social interactions to discuss their health statuses with people. Communicating about the cancer experience can open avenues for social support and enhance feelings of control over the disease (Badr & Taylor, 2006; Charmaz, 1991; Donovan-Kicken, Tollison & Goins, 2011). But it can also negatively impact survivors' positivity and how well they adapt to the experience (Badr & Taylor, 2006). Hence, a need for survivors to be proactive and set boundaries and the terms under which discussions about their experiences take place.

In this chapter, I focus on a phase in the ovarian cancer trajectory I term "owning the experience." This is the stage where survivors are in treatment and are trying to make sense of diagnosis and its implications for themselves and relational others. I examine communicative strategies survivors use to maintain inner balance and construct their own experiences amidst the uncertainties and identity challenges; that is, how they make sense of their experiences in their own ways. Owning the experience characterizes adjustment to diagnosis and treatments where survivors set the terms to define what their experiences mean to them and eliminate interfering messages and actions to manage their own uncertainties and those of others. This stage in the ovarian cancer trajectory brings to fore active roles survivors take in defining their experiences. While there are many things about the disease survivors cannot control (e.g., disease progression and treatment aftereffects), there are some things they can control, including allowing people's actions and attitudes to influence their experiences. I argue that this phase in the ovarian cancer trajectory is where women exhibit the most strength and courage by cooperating with science and medicine to take charge of their health and lives. Women's embodiments of strength and control challenge conventional views of the terms. Women may look weak and sick during treatments but that is when they are strongest and in control, contrary to general perceptions and portraits of strength.

It is important that survivors demonstrate control over their experiences because these experiences are theirs alone; thus, they are the best people to name and define these. Feminist scholars (e.g., Anzaldúa, 1992; Collins, 1986, 1990) argue that women and other marginalized groups have unique perspectives on their experiences which may be unavailable to people outside the group (i.e., epistemic knowledge/standpoint epistemology); thus, they have primary responsibility to define their own experiences and realities.

Dorothy Smith (1974) describes women as "native speakers" (p. 43) of their struggles and experiences as a result of having firsthand knowledge of these experiences. Oftentimes in the ovarian cancer context, survivors' sympathizers may rely on statistics and popular views about the disease to provide support and advice due to lack of personal experience with the disease. These popular notions about the disease often do not align with women's lived realities; hence, a need for survivors to boldly name their own experiences.

OWNING THE OVARIAN CANCER EXPERIENCE

For many women, owning the ovarian cancer experience begins shortly after diagnosis when they are recovering from the shock of diagnosis and trying to position themselves in relation to their new roles and identities (e.g., as sick people and receivers of care instead of caregivers). For others, it begins when treatments (which include combinations of surgery, chemotherapy, and/or radiation) are underway and they are sure they have the disease under control. In all, survivors deliberately made time to reflect on the diagnosis, treatments and the implications for their present and future selves. They aim to put the diagnosis into perspective and make sense of how they got where they are in order to forge a path forward. This is pertinent to understanding and expressing disconnects between their former and emerging identities; women are not who they used to be and are also not completely sure of who they are becoming. They are on the borderlines, in the middle. Given that diagnosis shook the core of their being, survivors need to "find" themselves again. In the process, some may distance themselves physically and/or mentally from people and belief systems. This may take place internally before manifesting externally where women involve relational others in the sense making process. Sense making at the internal level may include elements of self-advocacy, including carefully and deeply processing personal preferences, values, learned skills, and available support (Hagan & Donovan, 2013). It does not follow a predetermined pattern and may not be recognizable to women themselves. During this phase, people in survivors' social networks may not be aware of the internal meaning making taking place and may try hard to provide meaningful support. In response, survivors may play into standard scripts of support giving and receiving because they are not yet able to put into words the internal processes taking place. Survivors may put on strong fronts to coordinate their inner voices and protect loved ones; treatments may be grueling and prognosis may not be promising but they need to reassure themselves and those around them that there is light at the end of the tunnel.

Being thrusted into the category of the sick can be tough and terrifying for many ovarian cancer survivors partly because this is not a self-selected category and also because they are aware of the limitations and stigma associated with the sick identity (Atkins, 2016; Charmaz, 1999). Chronic illnesses challenge sufferers' identities in multiple ways, including limiting the ability to engage in prior activities and social roles (Martin, 2016). Many ovarian cancer survivors actively negotiate these identity and social role changes by managing seemingly contradictory messages and behaviors. Communication is central to how threats to identities are managed (Hecht, 1993; Martin, 2016). Survivors need stability and consistency within themselves and in their outside environments to go through treatments and beyond. They need to maintain a consistent narrative about their experiences, meaning that they need to negotiate and manage interferences.

To construct a coherent and consistent narrative about their experiences, some survivors may "force" themselves to look strong and healthy—a behavior that simultaneously challenges the "sick role" perspective and plays into normative views of women as selfless and natural caregivers (Sulik, 2007a). Others also may assume identities different from their usual character, including becoming docile and compliant. These may be women's responses to grueling treatments which weaken their bodies. Women harness inner strength to cooperate with treatments; active involvement in treatments becomes an avenue for women to assume control over an uncertain disease (Ferrell et al., 2003). It is a means for survivors to manage their own uncertainties and those of loved ones. Further, as part of constructing a consistent narrative, survivors may delay joining support groups and control the flow of information about the disease, including deciding not to inquire about other survivors' experiences with treatments. Women set these boundaries to manage their uncertainties, make meaning of their experiences in their own ways, and take attention from the illness (Brashers, 2001; Brashers et al., 2000; Miller, 2014). The process of owning the experience is influenced by survivors' age, level of available social support, stage of disease, treatment protocol, and recurrence status. The process is described in figure 3.1.

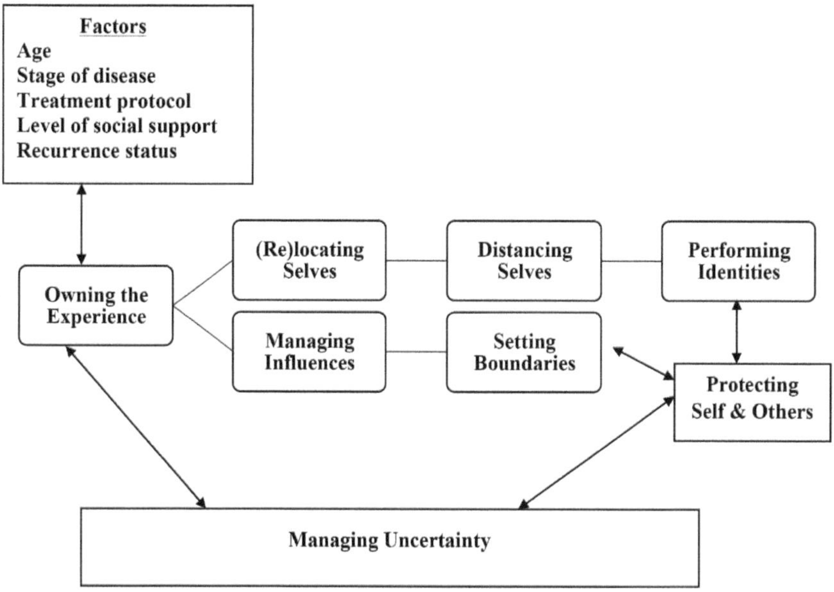

Figure 3.1. The Process of Owning the Ovarian Cancer Experience

(RE)LOCATING THE SELF

The process of owning the experience includes deliberate efforts by survivors to (re)locate the self in the ovarian cancer trajectory. Many survivors are unable to immediately grasp implications of diagnosis partly because of lack of knowledge about the disease (Gubar, 2012; Holmes, 2006; Reb, 2007). Some learn about the disease after diagnosis. Thus, while some are devastated by the diagnosis, others find it less surprising especially if they had symptoms that pointed to cancer (Ekman et al., 2004; Fitch et al., 2002; Reb, 2007). Regardless of how survivors receive a diagnosis, the immediate concerns of most of them relate to managing decisions about treatments and treatment side effects; reality of the diagnosis and prognosis begins to sink in when they are settled in treatments (Reb, 2007).

The period from diagnosis to the start of treatments proceeds quickly, leaving most survivors with no time to take a breath and make sense of everything (Ekman, Bergbom, Ekman, Berthold & Mahsneh, 2004). Amidst the roller-coaster of emotions following diagnosis, it is pertinent that survivors pause at a point to breathe, reflect on what is going on, and decide how to move forward. They need a mental pause to put things into perspective. The cancer experience is a process with a starting point (i.e., onset of symptoms and/or diagnosis); but it may not have an end for most people, particularly if there are recurrences and lingering treatment aftereffects (Salander, 2001). This is the situation for many ovarian cancer survivors.

(Re)locating the self also includes processing how and why survivors got cancer and how diagnosis and treatments may impact their lives, health, and the lives of loved ones. Some call this process meaning making, which is important to adapting to and coping with cancer (Fife, 1994) and to keeping hope alive (Bowes, Tamlyn & Butler, 2002). Meaning making is significant to preparing oneself psychologically for the "long haul." For instance, Andrea (43 years, stage III) explained that once treatment was underway and she was sure she had the disease under control, she and her "husband allowed [ourselves] one day of sadness just to get it all out. And from that moment on during my treatments I have really never cried." This "day of sadness" was a landmark moment in Andrea's ovarian cancer experience; she learned to breathe and to consciously process all that was going on. From that moment on, Andrea's perspective about her cancer journey changed; she determined what her experience would mean for herself and those in her social circle. Andrea had the support of her husband (and later, her best friend) to externalize the meaning making of her illness; but, up until that point she handled the process alone without expressing much of her feelings.

Distancing Selves

In the process of (re)locating themselves in the ovarian cancer experience and trying to make sense of diagnosis, some survivors may withdraw physically and/or mentally from people and/or belief systems. This is in an effort to reconcile who they were and who they are becoming—a need to reconcile their changing identities. It is also part of the process of seeking answers and justification for their health conditions. Withdrawing from social networks is different from the concept of communication avoidance where cancer patients and/or communication partners deliberately avoid discussing cancer for varied reasons (Caughlin, Mikucki-Enyart, Middleton, Stone, & Brown, 2011). The timing and nature of this distancing may differ for survivors depending on age, stage of disease, religious background, and available social support. Some women experience distancing during treatments, others experience it at the end of treatments, while others still experience it in the event of a recurrence.

For instance, Becca (57 years, stage III) explained why she distanced herself from God. She had symptoms which pointed to cancer and had hoped her fears would be disproved. When it turned out she had cancer, Becca was disappointed and needed to "think it through" with God. She said, "I was so annoyed with God; I was angry, disappointed, surprised and just could not believe God would put me through this. I kept saying 'this is not possible; God will never let this happen to me.' So when it happened, I was completely astonished and I went into total silence for a month." Like other survivors, Becca sought answers, which were not readily forthcoming. Questioning one's faith or God is part of the process of internal meaning making and women learning to reconstruct their worldviews and belief systems anew. Women may not expressly communicate their frustrations as God is not a physical being; but the act of demanding answers means that women are actively processing their diagnosis. Cancer survivors generally search for meaning through attribution (i.e., searching for answers), illusion (i.e., perceiving the situation different than what it is), positive reappraisal, and problem-focused coping (Lee et al., 2004; Coward & Kahn, 2005; Park, 2010; Skaggs & Barron, 2006). Searching for meaning is an active process that depends on one's existing worldviews, goals, and beliefs, among others (Thompson & Pitts, 1993), and it may be futile and distressing for most people (Kernan & Lepore, 2009).

In a similar vein, some survivors may distance themselves from friends and loved ones as part of the process of sense making. This can take the form of refusing visits from others or declining to take part in social events. This social distancing can stem from women's uncertainties about their lives and health. Survivors are walking in uncharted territories and need to be able to understand the course of that journey for themselves first before letting others in. They need to solidify their inner balance before they can open up their vulnerabilities to others. Survivors distancing themselves from other people can also be the result of side effects of treatments, including insomnia, pain, fatigue, nausea, depression, and medically-induced menopause. Survivors' identities are altered by treatments and side effects that they are unsure how society will receive and treat their emerging selves. For some survivors, this altered identity may include waned physical strength where they are unable to participate in activities they previously engaged in. The limitations treatments placed on women's physical bodies may cast doubts about their capabilities as mothers, wives, grandmothers, workers in the labor force, etc. They cannot tell if they will be mocked or genuinely cared for by others; it is hard to discern the motives of friends wanting to visit—whether it is out of concern or curiosity. Thus, to protect themselves and their emotions, which may be raw at that point in the cancer experience, some survivors distance themselves until their confidence levels rise to the point where they can withstand negativities from society. For instance, Patricia (67 years, stage III) explained, "I did not want to be around my grandchildren because in the past I was running around with them, playing football; but I was not that person anymore. I was a sitter, docile, and not cheerful." Patricia was still trying to find herself and make sense of the new identity forced on her by ovarian cancer; thus, she claimed the space she needed to re-know herself before she could reach out and have meaningful engagements with others. Patricia noted she also questioned the motives of friends who insisted on visiting despite her requests for them not to come. She explained, “I wonder if it is their curiosity as much as anything else. Did they want to see what kind of state I was in? What I looked like? Does it look like I would make it or was I on my deathbed? Sometimes that would come to mind, and maybe none of them had that idea but that’s life; we’re always curious about the odd one.” The effects of treatments on her physical body and identity impacted Patricia’s trust in people, the quality of her interpersonal relationships, and how well she availed herself of available social support. It got to a point where she feared she would lose her friends as she constantly refused their requests to visit. Atkins (2016) explains that effects of cancer and its treatments on survivors’ identities can affect their use of social support.

Along similar lines, survivors also may distance themselves from friends and loved ones in order to be “me again.” Many survivors receive great level of care and support from relational others—support that can sometimes overwhelm and negate survivors’ efforts to be independent and self-sufficient—the identities they avow. When social support undermines or interferes with survivors’ efforts to negotiate undesired identities (i.e., as sick people and receivers of care), it is construed negatively and challenged by women. Women actively negotiate when to draw a line between receiving support and interferences in their independence. This negotiation of role expectations and enactment of independence and self-care can be empowering and at the same time overwhelming. It can lead to identity crisis and role confusion for survivors, increase stress, and impact how they avail themselves of available support (Sulik, 2007a,b). For instance, Andrea explained she was unnerved by her mother’s overly protective attitude. She stated, “I had to distance myself [from my mother] for a little bit. She was calling 3–4 times a day asking, ‘Did you eat?’ ‘How are you feeling?’ ‘Did you get sick today?’ One day she came over and we were making dinner and every once in a while I would catch her staring at me and I said ‘mom, I am not dead yet; I am right here, stop staring at me.’ And she was like ‘sorry.’ So I had to distance myself from her.” Andrea needed consistency in her inner self and outside environment, consistency in how she perceived herself and was perceived by others. Her mother did not quite understand this because Andrea could not adequately communicate this, creating role conflicts. As observed by Deana Goldsmith (2009), interpersonal communication in the illness context can be both a source of uncertainty and anxiety as well as a resource for managing anxiety.

Reciprocally, some women also experience distancing from social networks. Friends may avoid survivors because they do not know how (or do not want) to deal with cancer. Cancer is still a scary word and for ovarian cancer, which has poor prognosis, people may not want to associate with the disease. People do not want to hear less-than-promising cancer stories (Gubar, 2012). For example, Christie (59 years, stage III) expressed her frustration with friends who avoided her because of a misconception that they had to talk about cancer each time they met. She said, "There have been very few people who have distanced themselves from me. I think they have this idea that when they see me, they have to talk about [my battle with ovarian cancer], which could not be more opposite." Patricia (67 years, stage III) also explained her experience with friends distancing themselves as follows: "I have friends that I have not heard from. I am thinking they probably did not know what to say. What do you say? I am sorry? They do not know how to respond." Similarly, Ruth (55 years, stage IV) noted how rejection from friends hurt her self-esteem, "I have friends, life-long friends, who walked away from me because they could not take it. And it hurts my heart. I was in a relationship; he walked away. And if that does not hurt your heart it beats the hell out of your self-esteem." Additionally, Lynn (60 years, stage II), who was terminal at the time of our interview, explained how her father could not stay in the same room with her because he had not yet come to terms with her impending death. She said, "There are some people that do not know how to deal with you because you are dying so they do not want to deal with you at all. My own father has a hard time dealing with me; he cannot stand being in the same room with me. It is easier for him to get up and go to the other room or go outside and do something than sit down and talk to me, because he cannot deal with my [impending] death." Death and dying are some of the difficult topics to communicate about in the cancer context. Cancer-related distress and fear of death can hinder effective communication between family members and cancer survivors (Caughlin, Mikucki-Enyart, Middleton, Stone, & Brown, 2011; Zhang & Siminoff, 2003). Some terminally-ill cancer survivors may want to openly discuss their impending deaths to disclose their last wishes; but family members may not be emotionally ready to accept the reality of losing a family member thus, avoid communicating about the topic. Some family members may also avoid talking about a relative's impending death to protect themselves and other family members, to keep hope alive, or because they feel they are not skilled (or lack efficacy) to discuss the topic (Caughlin et al., 2011).

Rejection from friends and family is not an uncommon experience for cancer survivors. Atkins (2016) found in her study on women cancer survivors that some relational others limited communication with survivors following a cancer diagnosis. Differences in treatment preferences and perceptions about whether survivors were responsible for their health predicaments are some of the reasons for the distancing survivors experience from their social networks. Distancing or "silence" is a way to manage some of the differing perceptions about treatments and communicating about cancer-related fear and distresses (Atkins, 2016; Zhang & Siminoff, 2003). And, as examples in this chapter illustrate, distancing and rejection survivors experience are multifaceted. Distancing can stem from relational others' fear of their own mortality and also as a result of survivors not wanting social company because of issues related to identity and uncertainties.

Facing rejection and distancing can be one of the hardest experiences for survivors to communicate about. This portrays sources of survivors' uncertainties and fears as both internal and external, with the external factors exerting additional toll on what women may be experiencing internally. It also points to the reality of the shared experience of cancer; people who do not carry the disease in their physical bodies also experience disease-related pain, and distancing may be their way of communicating this pain. This is exemplified in Andrea's cancer experience when her in-treatment body scared away one of her children. She said, "My middle kid handled [my diagnosis and treatments] the worst. He got more angry than sad. He wouldn't come home and stay with me. He would be around me but it was like he was afraid to see me." While many survivors are understanding of the reaction of loved ones, the situation nonetheless can be stressful and heighten women's uncertainties about their health. This distancing from/of others is crucial in helping women locate themselves in the whole experience, further providing the drive to "own" their experiences. Women come to the realization that this is *their* life, experience, and ordeal and they have to make it their *own*.

PERFORMING IDENTITIES

Distancing themselves and their experiences in an effort to protect themselves and loved ones can lead survivors to perform socially-sanctioned identities and roles to meet relational expectations. Identity is one's sense of self (i.e., a sense of who one is) that is communicated to others. We come to understand and negotiate who we are through social relationships and we also enact our identities through communication in social interactions (Jung & Hecht, 2004). Communication scholars have explained that identity and social roles and relations are intertwined, shaping each other through communication (Jung & Hecht, 2004). Identity resides in the self as well as in social relations—as seen in the four identity frames identified in the communication theory of identity (i.e., personal, enacted, relational, and communal; Hecht, 1993; Jung & Hecht, 2004).

Diagnosis with an illness threatens one's identity such that avowed and ascribed identities have to be renegotiated and managed. Identity negotiation is ongoing and constantly changing throughout the illness trajectory (i.e., patient, survivor, or caregiver; Little, Paul, Jordens & Sayers, 2002; Miller, 2015). In the event of an illness, there may be reversal of social relational roles where survivors become receivers of care instead of caregivers, for instance; or communication of roles and identities become contradictory resulting in identity gaps (Jung & Hecht, 2004). For example, contradictions between the personal and relational frames of identity, according to the communication theory of identity, occur when relational others see survivors through the emerging identity frame of a "sick person" contrary to survivors' desire to be seen as healthy and through the lens of their "old selves." While these interpenetrations of identities (Jung & Hecht, 2004) can help survivors make sense of their emerging identities, they can also present challenges especially if these role and identity negotiations coincide with efforts to manage uncertainties about the disease. Because of these issues and because some identities are more clear-cut (e.g., patient) than others (e.g., survivor), identity negotiation becomes difficult for many people affected by illnesses. For instance, Miller (2015) observed that cancer survivors and their partners experienced intrapersonal (i.e., internal) identity challenges as a result of identity shifts as well as interpersonal identity challenges arising from difficulties communicating preferred identities to relational others. Similarly, ovarian cancer and treatments can threaten survivors' identities as mothers, wives, partners, carers, and daughters because social roles performances in relational contexts shape survivors' identities and are in turn shaped by survivors' identities (Jung & Hecht, 2004). In this vein, this book suggests that performance of identities can occur in medical and relational contexts; in the former as survivors interact with health care providers and the medical system and in the latter as they interact with family and friends.

In the medical context, survivors' behaviors bear resemblance to expectations of the sick. Faced with an uncertain diagnosis and future where the only certainty is the hope that treatments will kill cancer cells, women cooperate with medical and scientific expertise and exert control over the disease through compliance. This means they rigidly follow tough treatment regimens and adhere to medical recommendations; active involvement in treatments becomes a means to take control over the disease (Ferrell et al., 2003). Enduring harsh treatments becomes a safety net for survivors and the medical facility becomes their safe zone. Women feel secure in the medical setting, a setting that concomitantly is an unfamiliar territory; they feel safe at the hospital but at the same time feel they do not belong there. Patricia (67 years, stage III) explained she felt "like a fish out of water" and "very vulnerable" while in treatment and said she assumed a different identity during treatments. She stated, "When I received news of my diagnosis until I was done with treatments, I became very docile and very quiet and compliant and would pretty much do whatever anyone told me to do. I changed into a totally different person." Patricia was uncertain about her health and life at that point and acted consistent with normative expectations of the ill—she took on the sick role (Charmaz, 1999). Trust in her doctor, lack of technical expertise about the disease and treatments, and harsh treatment side effects intersected to determine how she demonstrated agency over her experience—

by seemingly giving over control. Ironically, Patricia's behavior and sick-role performance earned commendation from her physician who described her as a "good patient." In a study about cancer survivors' constructions of their bodies across the cancer trajectory, Parton and colleagues (2017) find that women adopt body-as-object positions when in treatments where the body is seen as an object under the control of the medical system to be treated. With this mindset, women embody treatments passively as "something that happened *to* [them], without a sense of choice in the process" (p. 51), consistent with biomedical discourses about the body. But, there are some counter-experiences where women adopt body-as-subject positions of control and choice over their experiences.

Similarly, with awareness that one would feel sick and tired during cancer treatments, Andrea (43 years, stage III) questioned if she was acting in accordance with the ill/cancer identity when she did not experience any of the expected side effects of treatments. The pervasive ovarian cancer narrative (i.e., advanced disease, grueling treatments, and/or recurrences; Gubar, 2012; Holmes, 2006) was the framework available to Andrea to understand her own experience. She looked for evidence in her physical body relative to normative descriptions of the disease and finding none, she questioned her embodiment of the disease. She asked, "why am I not reacting that way? Am I supposed to feel sick? If I'm not feeling sick, is [the chemotherapy] not working?" It was later that Andrea embraced her own physical responses to treatments, using these to frame her illness narrative. Based on cultural assumptions about suffering (that it has to be purposeful), many cancer survivors consider excruciating treatments more effective (Bell, 2009). The sick role identity is not consistent for people affected with chronic illnesses. While an illness such as cancer can clearly demarcate the social identity groups people belong to (i.e., as sick people or healthy people; Charmaz, 1999) sometimes this distinction is not clear-cut, leaving ill people in the middle, on the borderlines, as was the case with Andrea.

In the context of social relationships, as well, survivors face the challenge of managing effects of treatments as well as negotiating altering identities. In this space, survivors' negotiations of their changing identities occur on both internal and external levels. The internal aspect appears to be the most difficult part of survivors' illness experiences because it is hard to express and communicate. In line with relational expectations, women may act "strong," "healthy," and "normal" in an effort to make diagnosis and treatments less severe for loved ones and also to cling to previously valued identities. They do not want to disrupt the social and relational orders of their families: they want their children to be kids, partners to have a life apart from cancer (e.g., keep golfing and fishing), and for parents to still feel they have capable (not sick) daughters. They want life to be normal for those around them. Seeing to it that this happens takes extra effort on the part of survivors as some "force" themselves to look healthy and normal—it is hard to put up a performance. This identity performance can be subtle where survivors do not disclose every tiny detail of how they are feeling, use general language to express symptoms, or deflect attention from themselves onto other things. For example, Nora (59 years, stage II) noted, "I would not tell [my parents] a whole lot about what was going on because I know how bad it hurts them. I felt bad that I was the one who was ill so I tried to protect them." Survivors feel responsible for their own well-being in addition to the well-being of loved ones and experience guilt when their illness seemingly impacts the welfare of those they love. Given their positions in the family and society and the roles they play as carers and nurturers, survivors feel compelled to continue performing these roles even when there are ill. Survivors' practice of selflessness in the context of illness has been discussed in the literature (e.g., Atkins, 2016; Sulik, 2007a).

Similarly, survivors who do not have partners or children also perform expected identities as survival mechanisms: they need a sense of inner balance to fight the disease. Performing expected relational roles and/or identities and distancing the self and experiences influence each other and together, they add to the nuances of the lived experience of ovarian cancer.

Threat to their identities as mothers are some of the difficult challenges ovarian cancer survivors negotiate. It can be difficult particularly if survivors' children are young and at home to witness diagnosis and treatments. In the same space where survivors can express their frustrations and fears, they also must express and embody support and care for young children. This can be tough and conflicting. As explained in chapter 2, it is a struggle for some women to use the word "cancer" to explain their diagnosis to young children. Andrea explained how she negotiated the threat posed to her identity as a mother by ovarian cancer. She tried for the entire time she was in treatment not to look sick in the presence of her children. She said, "I did not want my children to see me sick; so I never allowed it. I made sure that I got up every day and took a shower and put makeup on. It was hard but I did it. It was tough. There was only two times of the last nine months that I could not get up; the rest of the time, I forced myself to get up." Ellen (42 years, stage I) also mentioned that she performed being a mother and unifier of her family. She stated, "I found that the stronger I was on the outside the calmer things were with the people around me. So I had the tendency to be strong for everybody." Gena (79 years, stage III) also stated performing "strong" as a way of reclaiming her identity supposedly lost to ovarian cancer. She remarked, "once I was through with the treatments, I wanted to prove to myself and the world that I was still Gena. I always made sure I looked good because I did not want people to think, 'oh, she has cancer, look at how she looks.'" Performing identities is not only to protect people in their social networks, including spouses, children, parents, and friends; it was also necessary to forge inner balance and manage uncertainties about their health.

Evident in the foregoing discussion are reasons why ovarian cancer survivors perform socially sanctioned identities during the illness trajectory. Survivors are thrown into roles they are not prepared for, roles they may not choose if given the chance. Performing identities of a mother, wife, and so on requires that women look "strong," "healthy" and "normal"; and it is a way for them to protect their loved ones, avoid being treated differently, cement their hope of beating the disease, and reclaim their identities. For most survivors, it is pertinent that how they feel and act in the face of the uncertainties of the disease match how they are treated by those in their social networks; hence, a need to "perform" in order to score the desired reaction from relational others. This supports previous research findings that cancer survivors perform identities to seek validation for their preferred identities (Donovan-Kicken et al., 2011; Ekman et al., 2004) and to protect their loved ones (Atkins, 2016; Zhang & Siminoff, 2003). It is also to manage the uncertainties associated with the disease (Hipkins et al., 2004; Lockwood-Rayermann, 2006) and to foster an inner sense of security.

Ovarian cancer survivors' performance of socially sanctioned identities and roles is consistent with normative gender expectations. Women's age and stage of disease are not significant factors in whether women performed expected roles and identities. While cancer survivors sometimes become "gender conscious" and defy gender role expectations by putting their interests first, at other times they play into gender expectations they seek to break free from (Sulik, 2007a, p. 303). They struggle to provide care work for the self (Sulik, 2007b). It is a fluid performance dictated by context, disease, and individual characteristics.

MANAGING INFLUENCES

As part of making sense of the cancer experience in their own ways, survivors set parameters to define what their experiences mean for themselves and others. Managing influences describes steps survivors take to determine how their experiences unfold, solidify their inner voices, and minimize interferences. Survivors are in the process of adjusting to diagnosis and treatments and need consistency in the messages of hope they recount to themselves and other messages in their environments. They actively manage messages, behaviors, and thoughts that interfere with how they want their experiences to unfold. Survivors are aware negativities and misconceptions about ovarian cancer can exacerbate an already difficult experience for them; thus, they actively filter out negative influences as much as possible. They do this by choosing when and how much to know about the disease, when and whether or not to join a support group, and how much of their experiences is disclosed on social media. Survivors set these boundaries to protect their own lived experiences and that of other survivors and to regain the control seemingly lost to cancer. Below, I discuss some of the communicative strategies survivors use to set boundaries around their experiences.

Setting Boundaries

Many survivors consider a diagnosis with ovarian cancer tough enough that it may be unwarranted to add additional stresses by knowing details of their particular cancer cell, for example, or the specifics of treatments. Depending on their psychological capabilities, survivors may prefer not to know these details or choose to receive this information in bits. Choosing to approach their experiences in this manner does not mean survivors are in denial of their diagnosis; this is their individual preference for managing their experiences. For instance, Nora (59 years, stage II) chose not to know her cancer cell type and the drugs she was being treated with to prevent information overload and to direct conversation around her illness. Whenever she was conversing with others and they asked about her cancer cell type she told them she did not know to silence speculations about her prognosis and to avoid being pitied. Kylie (65 years) also did not ask about her prognosis and stage of cancer for fear that information might interfere with her psychological preparedness to fight the disease. She wanted to beat the odds, and actively determined what information she needed and which she did not need to achieve that goal. She remarked, "My whole philosophy was to fight and it did not really sink in to me that I only had 30% chance of survival. I did not even remember [the doctor] saying [I had 30% chance of survival] until after I was declared cancer-free and then all those memories came back." Similarly, Mercy (58 years, stage I) explained she did not inquire about the standard treatment for ovarian cancer because she wanted to experience treatment her own way; she wanted her experience to be her own. She stated, "When I was going through chemotherapy, I did not want to hear other people's experiences; I just wanted to go into it blind and experience whatever was going to happen. I wanted it to unfold for me personally. I did not know how many treatments people typically have; I did not know that I was having that much chemo. I just did not want to know."

Significantly, living with a recurrent disease contributes to how survivors introduce and enforce boundaries around their experiences. Recurrences are not the disease progression course survivors anticipate when they are first diagnosed; they expect to deal with the disease once and never have to worry about it again. Thus, recurrences bring disappointment, dashed hope, and increased uncertainty. The more the disease recurs the more important it is for survivors to control how much information about their experiences is shared with distal others, particularly through social media. At this point in the illness experience, survivors are aware the disease can claim their lives; thus, they want their experiences to be personal where they share details of their illnesses only with close friends and family members. Survivors set these boundaries to sustain their sense of control over the disease, honor their memories in the event that they pass away, and protect other survivors who are still battling the disease.

Others also set boundaries around their experiences as an identity management strategy (Martin, 2016). Survivors living with recurrent ovarian cancer may be dealing with the disease for years unending (e.g., five or eight years); thus, it is possible for the disease to take over their identity. To change this and manage their conflated identities, some survivors put their ovarian cancer survivor identity in the background to refocus public attention on other aspects of their lives they want to be known and remembered for. They do this by referencing the disease less frequently during interactions and selectively disclosing symptoms they are experiencing to maintain their prior identities and to avoid having to deal with other people's feelings (Charmaz, 1999). For instance, Esther (48 years, stage III), who was living with recurrent disease, narrated how she managed her presence online as follows:

> I do not share my story and what is going on [on social media] because I do not want anybody to pity me. So often people hear stage III-C ovarian cancer and they go, 'oh, she is a goner'; 'oh, poor thing, she is gone.' Another reason is as a survivor, I have gone online and searched other people's pages and lots of them have died. That is hard especially if you are newly diagnosed and you are trying to find women who have survived and you find that they were really active and posting and then nothing and a family member comes in to say they have passed away. So I figured if I start a Caring Bridge[1] page and I die it must be hard for someone to see.

Moreover, survivors set boundaries by controlling messages and behaviors around their experiences to manage their uncertainties. At this point in the illness trajectory, survivors have significant knowledge about ovarian cancer to be uncertain about the future, their health, and the impact treatments can have on their identities and on relational others. It is important for many of them to not make their fears public because that can potentially contradict how they carry themselves and the strength they show in the face of adversity. Survivors are aware that recurrent disease may mean imminent death; but for them, succumbing to the disease does not mean they did not "survive" it. Thus, they made it their responsibility to protect/safeguard memories they have created for and with others. Previous research suggests that cancer survivors control information to regain some of the control lost to the disease (Charmaz, 1991; Donovan-Kicken et al., 2011) and to manage illness-related uncertainties (Babrow & Matthias, 2009; Brashers, Goldsmith, & Hsieh, 2002; Miller, 2014).

The examples presented in this chapter demonstrate how ovarian cancer survivors simultaneously challenge and reify gender role expectations. When necessary, survivors claim needed space to independently process their illness experiences. At the same time some of them feel entitled to provide care and protect relational others—gender role negotiations that occur throughout the illness trajectory (Sulik, 2007a,b). By setting boundaries to manage uncertainties, negotiate altering identities, and determine the cancer experience in their own ways, ovarian cancer survivors position themselves as active participants in the process of owning their experiences (Charmaz, 1991). Survivors actively shape their own meaning making of the disease, naming what counts and what does not.

NOTE

1. Caring Bridge is an online support platform where cancer patients and survivors share their experiences and update friends and loved ones on their health statuses. Users create journals to give updates on their health; loved ones are notified when there is an update and they can comment to provide support. See: https://www.caringbridge.org/how-it-works.

Chapter Four

Becoming an Ovarian Cancer Survivor

Managing Uncertainty and Survivor's Guilt

> *When I was done [with treatment] and put in remission, that scared me more than the whole time being in treatment because I knew the cancer was being killed off because I was in treatment. And then you stop [treatment] and you go, "well, now what? Is [the cancer] going to come back? Where is it going to come back at?" It's a guessing game.*
>
> *Andrea, 43 years, stage III*

The period following end of active treatment is critical to the overall health and quality of life of cancer survivors (Arnold, 1999; Garofalo et al., 2009). Quality of life for many survivors is generally low at this stage because of uncertainties about health, heightened stress about returning to "normal" life, and experiences with treatment side effects, including insomnia, fatigue, medically-induced menopause, and altered sexuality (Duffey-Lind et al., 2006; Garofalo et al., 2009; Knobf, 2007; McKenzie & Crouch, 2004). It is at this phase that losses suffered during treatments, including loss of hair, strength, or body parts are communicated, negotiated, and dealt with outside the health care setting (Hewitt, Greenfield, & Stovall, 2006). This phase in the cancer trajectory merits increased research attention because survivors' responses to diagnosis, treatments, and transition to survivorship are impacted by individual as well as societal factors and have implications for public perceptions about cancer.

Andrea's reflection (quoted above) on ending active treatment for ovarian cancer shows the uncertainties many cancer survivors face. She is a 43-year-old mother of three who went aggressively after the disease with nine weeks of chemotherapy, a radical hysterectomy during her six weeks off, and then another nine weeks of chemotherapy. Andrea, like many women affected by ovarian cancer, was anxious about going into medical remission after enduring months of treatments and becoming used to and, somehow, trusting treatments to get rid of the cancer cells. Once treatments were over, then what? Even though Andrea anticipated the end of treatments, she became vulnerable and ill-prepared to face life without/after treatments. This uncertainty about the future makes women like Andrea almost wish treatments never end because being in treatment and feeling worn-out provides assurance that they are actively fighting the disease. What does it mean to be an ovarian cancer survivor? How does end of treatment contribute to the process of becoming a survivor? What are the factors that influence the process for women? What roles do support groups (and systems) play in cancer survivorship? These are questions I explore in this chapter.

This chapter examines the *process* of ovarian cancer survivorship by examining sources of uncertainty in survivors, how uncertainties are communicatively managed, and factors contributing to survivors' constructions of their lived experiences. My aims include centering survivors' voices in the ovarian cancer survivorship narrative, illuminating concerns and stressors survivors experience at the end of treatment, and suggesting ways to tailor intervention and support services to better serve survivors. I argue that every woman affected by ovarian cancer is a survivor, in line with the National Coalition for Cancer Survivorship's (NCCS) definition of a cancer survivor. But, I suggest also that the process of survivorship becomes intentional at the end of active treatment when control over their health is somewhat back in women's hands. The transition from a cancer patient to a cancer survivor is a long, rough process, spanning months or years; it does not happen overnight. It involves conscious and subtle work by women and others in their social networks. For example, Kylie (65 years old) stated she "struggled" for years to become a cancer survivor and that "my struggle with becoming a cancer survivor was longer and far more intense than fighting cancer." Kylie's struggle was both physical and psychological. Cancer survivorship is ongoing, beginning with diagnosis; hence, it is appropriate to study it as a process. Unlike active treatments which have specific start and end periods, survivorship is enduring. Thus, crucial as the treatment phase is, even more crucial is the phase when women are no longer in treatment and have to navigate life without any roadmap or self-help book.

The process of survivorship differs for each woman depending on her stage in the post-treatment experience: some women are out of treatment for a long time (i.e., 17 years) while others recently finished treatment (i.e., four months); some have not experienced any recurrences while others have multiple recurrences. For each woman, then, the process of becoming a survivor is deeply personal and involves sorting through life at different paces and phases depending on age, socioeconomic status, level of available social support, and treatment aftereffects. For instance, women at the high end of the social and economic ladder may not experience some of the financial stresses other survivors face, and women who do not have lingering treatment aftereffects (such as neuropathy) are able to get their lives back together relatively quicker than those who experience these aftereffects. For most women, the process begins at the end of active treatments.

ENDING TREATMENTS

Finishing active treatments can be a difficult time in the ovarian cancer experience. It is a period filled with mixed emotions, including excitement, relief, hope, and optimism on the one hand and fear and uncertainty on the other. Women are "thrilled," "happy," and "thankful"; but can also be "scared" and "concerned" to be finishing treatments. They are thrilled their bodies are getting a reprieve from grueling treatments; that they are no longer "poisoned" by medications meant to save their lives; that their lives are no longer under the control of drugs and physicians; that they do not have to play the sick role anymore—in short, women are happy to have their lives back. However, they are also worried about the disease recurring because of acute awareness of the possibility. Advanced epithelial ovarian cancer has a high recurrence rate (Schink, 1999). These mixed feelings produce uncertainties in women about their lives, health, and the disease. Uncertainties can sometimes be so great they can overshadow joy at finishing treatments. Uncertainty occurs "when an event cannot be adequately structured or categorized because sufficient cues are lacking"; or when individuals cannot determine outcomes of situations because of insufficient cues to make such prediction (Mishel & Braden, 1987, p. 48).

Uncertainty management theory (UMT; Brashers et al., 2000; Brashers, 2001) and problematic integration theory (PI; Babrow, 1992, 2001) help explain uncertainties cancer survivors experience. PI theory posits that people form different probabilistic orientations (i.e., "associational webs of understanding that we form through more or less thoughtful engagement with the world;" Babrow, 2001, p. 560) and evaluative orientations toward their experiences. When there are difficulties integrating probabilistic and evaluative orientations, people experience different forms of problematic integration (including uncertainty). Further, PI theory distinguishes between foci (topics or issues) and forms (nature, sources, or reasons) of uncertainty. It stresses, however, that foci and forms of uncertainty are fundamentally interdependent and contextual; thus, efforts to manage[1] or cope with uncertainty are contextual (Babrow, 2001; see also Brashers, 2001). It recognizes ontological and epistemological forms/meanings of uncertainty; the former being uncertainty emanating from beliefs about indeterminate nature of the world whereas the latter is uncertainty relating to recognition of limits of our knowledge (i.e., sufficiency or validity of knowledge; Babrow, 2001). The forms of uncertainty (or problematic integrations in general) are fluid and interrelated such that initial problematic integrations can transform into different PIs (Babrow, 2001; Babrow & Matthias, 2009). For instance, uncertainty an ovarian cancer survivor may have about possibility of disease recurrence can change into uncertainty about financial security when she realizes she will be paying treatment costs for a long time. Further, this uncertainty can transform into a group concern when other survivors share the woman's concerns. PI theory also explains that because uncertainty has multiple meanings, managing levels of uncertainty is not the only means to managing uncertainty. Uncertainty can be managed by reappraising/reevaluating the object of uncertainty, accepting the status quo, or reframing uncertainty as an opportunity for growth. The theory stresses centrality of communication to uncertainty (and PI broadly) experiences (Babrow, 1992, 2001; see also Brashers, 2001).

Similarly, UMT (Brashers et al., 2000; Brashers, 2001) considers uncertainty a ubiquitous human experience, particularly in the illness context, that is managed (i.e., increased, decreased, or maintained) using communication behaviors. Brashers and colleagues (2000) explain that how uncertainty is appraised (i.e., as a danger, opportunity, or chronic condition) and the associated emotional reactions (positive, negative, or neutral) influence strategies used to manage uncertainty (e.g., information seeking or avoidance, reappraisal, adaptation, or seeking social support to increase, maintain or decrease uncertainty). In the health and illness context, unspecified illness cause and/or symptoms, unpredictable treatment outcomes, and conflicting information about treatment options can produce uncertainty about "financial well-being, the social reactions of others, and future changes in health status" (Brashers, 2001, p. 480).

Uncertainties ovarian cancer survivors experience stem partly from awareness of possible disease recurrence (emanating from unpredictable nature of disease). They are aware the disease may recur but do not know for certain when this will happen; there is constant fear of what to expect next, when (not if) the disease will recur, and where it will come back at. This creates uncertainties about women's health as they leave active medical care, and makes communication about their experiences, particularly at the end of treatments, forward-looking; they talk about and plan for what is next (i.e., the future) when they are in the now. They have to grapple with both now and the future and learn to be good at being hopeful in the midst of uncertainties. This juggling of concurrent and opposite feelings and realities portrays women as proactive; but also shows their discomfort with the uncertainties. Many of them appraise uncertainties as a threat that needs to be reduced (Brashers, 2001).

Andrea explained, "Do I think I will get cancer again? Probably. I think I will get it again. I do not know if it will be in my breast or somewhere else." Andrea did not undermine her chances of having cancer again; her BRCA gene mutation puts her at an increased risk of cancer. Andrea said she tried not to focus on the possibility of a recurrence because she had no control over that. Mercy (58 years, stage I) also mentioned she was aware of chances of her cancer recurring; but felt she had some time before starting to worry about that. She said, "Because I just finished chemotherapy I do not think it is going to recur right away. I feel like I have some time before I have to worry about it recurring again. But obviously I am very concerned because I know I have a 50% chance of recurrence." Women do not deny chances of the disease recurring; they are informed and educated about that. But since a recurrence is out of their control they adapt to it and focus on things they can control, including closely monitoring their diets and physical exercise patterns. Women's fear of a recurrence is connected to the nature of ovarian cancer, including its nonspecific symptoms, late diagnosis, and high recurrence and morality rates. There is no guarantee of cure after long and grueling treatments for the disease; and nonspecific symptoms provide no "safety signals" that the disease will not recur (Ekman et al., 2004; Howell et al., 2003; Hipkins, Whitworth, Tarrier & Jayson, 2004; Ozga et al., 2015; Reb, 2007).

In this context, then, time away from treatments becomes essential to how women communicatively manage uncertainties. Women who recently finished treatment openly communicate about their uncertainties because they are certain they have the disease under control (at least for now); the odds are in their favor. This is also true for women who have not experienced any recurrences. But the more recurrences women experience, the more private they become with their uncertainties about their health statuses, probably because conditions of their physical bodies communicate their failing health states such that it becomes redundant for women to restate the obvious. Nora (59 years, stage II) explained, "The more the cancer comes back, the more you become a little inward because at that point, it becomes extremely personal."

PUTTING THE PIECES TOGETHER

Once active treatments are over, women direct their attention toward getting back to "normal" life. The intensity of treatments necessitates that survivors put their lives (e.g., travels and work) on hold in order to focus and manage immediate side effects.[2] This is because, as explained by Kylie (65 years old), "You cannot deal with [ovarian cancer] as it happens to you. When I was dealing with my chemotherapy, I was trying to deal with how to live today; I did not have time to deal with anything else." Treatments are usually back-to-back with a few breaks in-between for women to catch a breath; they require everything women have, including their strength, attention, interests—their very lives. Women, thus, attend to immediate needs (e.g., food to eat for the day, getting enough rest, and getting to the next treatment) and leave larger issues (e.g., finances) until treatments are over. However, women soon realize they do not have to deal with only the anticipated issues but other unforeseen ones as well and that the path to survivorship is not clear-cut. There are no explicit rules to help navigate life after treatments; there are no sureties and blueprints. During treatments, survivors are certain they are actively battling the disease, but this sense of security diminishes when treatments end. Also, survivors have constant access to high-level medical and social support during treatments, but these forms of support recede once active treatments are over, leaving them feeling vulnerable, lost, scared, and uncertain about the future (Arnold, 1999; Duffey-Lind et al., 2006; Garofalo et al., 2009; Hewitt et al., 2006; Knobf, 2007; Lethborg, Kissane, & Sullivan, 2000; McKinley, 2000; Mishel & Braden, 1987; Reb, 2007). For example, Mercy (58 years old, stage I) stated, "The difficult thing is what your life is like afterwards; losing your job and trying to figure out insurance and issues about disability. It is the afterwards that you do not know. Nobody tells you that." Mercy was surprised by the challenges she needed to grapple with post-treatment, including disability (e.g., neuropathy), job loss, financial difficulties, sexual health issues, and weight gain. These challenges, added to treatment side effects they have to manage, can put women into silence, literally and figuratively speaking.

These challenges are unexpected for many survivors and can create uncertainties about the future (employment-, finance-, and relationship-wise). Because of severe neuropathy, Mercy was not sure she could return to work. She said, "Companies cannot hold your job forever. I'm not sure I can work because I have a hard time talking and a hard time walking." Similarly, effects of treatments on her sexual self-concept created doubts in Ruth (55 years old, stage IV) about the possibility of a romantic relationship. She explained, "I feel so deformed and so ugly; I hate looking at my body in the mirror. I have no interest in having a relationship with a man. I would love to get married but I do not see it in my future. If I cannot stand to look at myself in the mirror, I cannot even imagine a man would."

Navigating Financial Stressors

Changes women make in their work-life to accommodate treatments, including working part-time or taking early retirement, significantly affect their finances. Cost of treatments and out-of-pocket insurance co-pays also take huge financial tolls that support from social security disability and social networks may not alleviate. This leaves women in financial "holes" many of them doubt recovering from, producing uncertainties about their financial security. For example, Andrea explained she had incurred about half a million dollars in medical expenses. To Andrea, there was a price to life in that finance played a huge role in her ovarian cancer treatments and survivorship experience. She was alive but would have to pay the cost of living probably for the rest of her life. Ruth also explained her situation as follows: "I make very little money every month since I have had this sickness. I am lucky if I make $300–$400 a month; and that is to buy grocery and other things. I have had to file bankruptcy; they foreclosed [my house]. I now live in the basement in the home of my sister and her husband." Ruth was living with recurrent ovarian cancer, her partner left upon her diagnosis, she was not employed, and financial struggles appeared to be a consistent aspect of her experience. Financial stresses brought on by the disease made it impossible for Ruth to follow medical recommendation to eat healthy, heightening uncertainty about her health. She stated, "The doctor would say 'I want you to lose weight; I want you to eat more fresh vegetables and fruits.' Yeah, really? When I have $100 a month for grocery, I am going to buy pasta. What do you want me to do?" Similarly, Chelsea (56 years, stage I) explained she constantly "fights" with her insurance company over unpaid medical bills. She said, "insurance companies expect everybody to have family and for the family to jump in and take care of things; but not everybody does have family. I have family but they are all deceased." Also, Mercy echoed similar frustrations when she stated that "every day a mail comes in I am like 'am I going to have a crazy afternoon or a quiet afternoon?' because I am dealing with health care bills that have come in." As these examples demonstrate, lack of social support complicates survivors' financial uncertainty experiences. Even though financial support is considered unwanted because of the potential face-threat (Floyd & Ray, 2016), an awareness of lack of this support can produce uncertainty in survivors about the future and financial security.

On the other hand, strong support systems help women appraise financial fallouts from treatments positively and consequently manage uncertainties these produced. Support resources ameliorate financial fallouts from treatments. For instance, Andrea received tremendous financial support from her family and friends; over 700 people showed up for her fundraiser. Andrea and her husband were financially stable and she was able to put her "house in a trust so that if something would have happened to me my children can have a home to grow up in." Thus, even though debt from treatments produced uncertainty about her financial security, Andrea knew she had support to fall on. Andrea also received strong emotional support from her family members, who switched to organic foods and shaved their heads to show solidarity. This support (partly because of shared relational expectations and mutual interdependence) was instrumental in helping Andrea appraise and manage issues creating uncertainty, exemplifying theorizing about relational interdependence and illness (Goldsmith, 2009; Miller & Caughlin, 2013; Zhang & Siminoff, 2003). It also points to the interconnectedness between women's health and the health of their families (Dorgan, Duvall, Hutson & Kinser, 2013; Petersen, Kruckek & Shaffner, 2003), showing how this interconnectedness can be a great source of support during times of illness. Andrea described how she previously "didn't want to leave the house or put a scarf on because people are going to stare" but with the support of her family she began to go out "with pride; it's like the scars that I have are part of my journey."

Similarly, Patricia (67 years, stage III) mentioned that though it "cost a little more to pay out of pocket" for her treatments, she was able to afford it because "I put away a lot of money for retirement and I have a very good pension. I have never been worried about [the cost of treatments]." Patricia was divorced but she was financially stable going into treatment and had grown children who were doing well in life. Additionally, finance was not an issue for Esther (48 years, stage III), who was living with recurrent ovarian cancer. She explained, "For our 25th wedding anniversary I got a new diamond for my husband, and we would never have spent money like that; that would have been something we would have waited till we are married 50 years. But that may not happen." The diagnosis made Esther liberal with her spending given that the future was not guaranteed. This was part of her process of adapting to the chronic uncertainty about the future.

These examples point to significance of finance in the ovarian cancer context with critical implications for women's uncertainty experiences and conceptions of survivorship. The financial burden of cancer is aggravated for women with limited social and financial resources and those who cannot return to work due to recurrences and severe neuropathy, among others. Some survivors have limited social and financial buffers to begin with while others have strong support systems going into treatment, and this impacts their post-treatment experiences. This helps shed some light on recession of social support at the end of active cancer treatments (Arnold, 1999; Reb, 2007), making clear *why* this may not be the case for all survivors. It is important to understand this distinction to better conceptualize the support needs of ovarian cancer survivors at the end of treatment and help tailor individualized support and intervention programs.

Strong financial and support systems help cushion survivors against fallouts from treatments and increase their sense of security in the future; knowing they have support systems to depend on can help survivors appraise and react to illness-related uncertainties positively. For example, relational others (e.g., partners and children) switched diets alongside survivors and shaved their heads to show solidarity—communicative behaviors that helped validate women's experiences about living in altered bodies. However, women who lack adequate support usually handle treatment aftereffects (e.g., financial struggles) single-handedly; this can incapacitate their efforts to make dietary changes, for example, providing grounds for uncertainties about their health.

The crucial role of social networks in the health and illness context cannot be overstated (Brashers, Neidig & Goldsmith, 2004; Umberson & Montez, 2010). Whether enacted or not, social support can have positive impacts on physical and psychological health (Callaghan & Morrissey, 1993). With a few exceptions (e.g., Trivers, Patterson, Roland & Rodriguez, 2013), financial difficulties are often not acknowledged in mainstream cancer discourses as they contradict standard narratives of hope and optimism (Koczwara & Ward, 2014). This book suggests this needs to change and advocates for recognition of finance as a crucial aspect of the ovarian cancer experience.

It is important to recognize that while the physical tolls of treatments may be a reason why few ovarian cancer survivors open up about their experiences (Gubar, 2012), the psychological tolls, including financial hardships, also contribute to survivors' undesirability to publicly share their experiences. The majority of women I interviewed did not publicly discuss their financial struggles because of potential face-threats and because of conventional expectations of cancer survivors to live with gratitude (Little, Paul, Jordans, & Sayers, 2002; Zebrack, 2000). These expectations are consistent with popular constructions of breast cancer survivorship,[3] often associated with optimism, stoicism, and advocacy (Michel, 2014; Sulik, 2011), and can coerce ovarian cancer survivors into silence about the realities of their circumstances. Feminist scholars and others have denounced the undue pressure and stress these expectations put on survivors, arguing that differences in embodiments of the cancer experience should be embraced (Sulik, 2011). The excitement others feel about survivors' health progress can take up the space (and listening ears) survivors need to discuss their financial situations. When communication about such a sensitive topic is blocked, it takes a long time to rebuild trust and courage to broach the topic again. For instance, Mercy mentioned she had severe neuropathy which prevented her from returning to work and when she complained about her situation, her friend retorted, "what do you care? You're alive!" While this remark was intended to make Mercy feel better, it lacked sensitivity to Mercy's face, constricted communication about her experience, and affected her future support-seeking behaviors (see Burleson & Goldsmith, 1998). Mercy said from then on she only shared her experience with people who genuinely wanted to listen and she refrained from sharing specific details.

GOING PUBLIC

Another remarkable source of uncertainty was perceptions about benefits of support groups and other public awareness events. When women feel ready psychologically (i.e., they are "at the other side of the [cancer] experience") and consider events expedient, they utilize support groups, programs to teach medical students about ovarian cancer, fundraisers, and cancer walks to connect with other survivors. I focus on support groups here. Participation in support groups is not consistent across the board within and among women. Women who presently do not see a need for support groups may join one later and those who currently participate in some groups may withdraw at a future date. There are varied reasons and motivations why ovarian cancer survivors may (or may not) join support groups, including recurrence status, length of years living with disease, age, and available social support.

Women consider support groups a means to identify with the disease, draw strength and hope from other survivors, and process their experiences by talking it through with others. Considerations about whether or not to join support groups are not dependent on support survivors receive from relational others. Rather, it depends on evaluative benefits of support groups (determined by the individual) and how far away women are from treatments. Some survivors feel family members and close others do not understand their perspectives because they lack firsthand experience with the disease. But, other survivors can relate because of commonalities in experience. For instance, Kylie (58 years, stage I) explained she joined a support group because she "felt disconnected in a way. Nobody understood me and I felt only the support group members could understand because they can relate. Even though your family is very loving, they hear cancer-free and they are like 'oh okay, that is it.' Unfortunately, that is not it because your mind cannot go from a cancer patient to being a cancer-free person; it does not work that way." Differences in social expectations and actual experiences of disease can present barriers when communicating about the cancer experience (Miller, 2015) and can increase uncertainties in survivors. Other survivors also join support groups to be an encouragement to those recently diagnosed. This is their way of "paying it forward" and "showing" that the disease can be survived. These survivors use their lived experiences to help other women find their voices and positively appraise their experiences. As survivors help others to find their voices, their own understandings of their experiences are refined.

However, some survivors do not join support groups because of perceived non-beneficial outcomes (e.g., that support groups will be detrimental to their psychological well-being) or lack of logistics to attend group meetings. Among women in this category are younger survivors and those who recently completed treatment. Also, some may decide not to join support groups to manage uncertainties related to death and dying and to take control of their experiences. Problematic Integration theory (PI; Babrow, 1992, 2001) suggests that communication (or social interaction) is central to the experience and transformation of uncertainty (or problematic integration broadly). Because of high disease mortality rate, it is not uncommon for ovarian cancer survivors to witness deaths of support group members—an experience that can make the disease real for them and create uncertainties about their own mortality.

Facing Mortality

Many women I interviewed named exposure to death and dying a key source of uncertainty about their own health statuses. For instance, Christie (59 years, stage III) mentioned, "I have three very good friends who lost it to ovarian cancer. That affects your thinking and mortality because you realize it is right in front of you." Nora (59 years, stage II) also said, "In some ways the support group scared me because I would hear stories that were so horrible. I was doing okay; I was working and I did not want to think that [the cancer] could come back." Nora did not need reminders that her cancer could recur, but this was sometimes inevitable in a support group setting. As a safe space for people with common experiences, support groups are a place survivors turn to for reminders that the disease can be survived. However, because groups consist of survivors at various stages in the cancer journey there are no guarantees that discussions in the groups will only be what women want to hear. Others' life stories can help survivors put their own lived experiences into perspective but can also increase their uncertainties. Communication and experiences that may be offensive to some members may sound perfectly okay to others. Ruth (55 years, stage IV), explained her experience of loss in support groups and how that affected not only her own mortality by her views about forming relationships with support group members. She said,

> We had a lot of members that died. It is hard because you are with them and they are bearing their souls to you on an intimate level; you know what they have gone through and they also know what you have been through. You are even forging a friendship and puff, they are gone. And it starts again and then another one is gone. It is really hard because you see it more in an ovarian cancer group.

This goes to support the high mortality rate of ovarian cancer and its effects on relationship building in support groups.

Experiences in support groups suggests that women need to learn to balance and coordinate not only changes in their lives in the transition to survivorship but also differences in others' experiences of the disease. To become the survivor they want, women have to learn to quickly sort out encounters at support groups and other public events that are meaningful to their own lived experiences and leave out those that are counter-productive. They have to learn to communicate and build relationships in ways that support where they are at and where they want to get to in the cancer experience. This requires some level of psychological stamina. While each woman's situation is different and the experience of ovarian cancer is never the same for everyone, seeing the struggles of other survivors can send women on an imagination journey to figure out "what could be" of their future selves—a situation that can exacerbate uncertainty.

Feeling Guilty

In a similar vein, support groups (and other public events) provide avenues for women to appraise their experiences. Using the experiences of other survivors and normative constructions of the disease as yardsticks, women diagnosed at early stages (i.e., stages I and II) and those whose disease has not recurred become uncertain about legitimacy of their experiences and how other survivors (e.g., those diagnosed with advanced disease) will respond to them. These women feel "guilty" for not suffering enough. For instance, 20-year-survivor Pattie (38 years, stage III) explained, "Sometimes I feel guilty being a survivor because so many people have passed away." Lucy (60 years, stage I) also said, "I feel guilty saying I am a survivor. I only had three chemotherapy treatments and there are other women fighting for their lives. When I am in the general public, I do not really have a problem, but when I am among other [survivors], that is when I am hesitant to use the word "survivor." I feel that maybe I should have suffered a little more." Survivors who harbor these guilty feelings normally self-censor when communicating with fellow survivors, as an uncertainty management strategy. For instance, Juliet (59 years, stage II), a 12-year survivor whose disease had not recurred, stated being very guarded when talking in her support group in order not to hurt the feelings of other survivors and to not come across as self-righteous.

To better understand the concept of guilt in ovarian cancer survivorship, it is imperative to consider normative constructions of the disease (e.g., late diagnosis, grueling treatments, and recurrences) and of a cancer survivor (e.g., heroic and optimistic). Perceptions about ovarian cancer are influenced, to a large extent, by its not-so-pleasant public representations (see Holmes, 2006) and limited "happily-ever-after" survival narratives (Gubar, 2012, p. 23). Martha Holmes (2006) argues that lack of "public faces" on the disease (in terms of celebrities who have had the disease) and metaphors of "silent killer," and "whispering" contribute to limit ovarian cancer's public visibility. Public discourse around the disease often takes place following the death of a public personality or someone close to them (e.g., Angelina Jolie). Put simply, the disease is portrayed as un-survivable. In terms of who qualifies as a cancer survivor, popular conceptions imply survivors are those cured from cancer and that the survivor label is earned through fighting and beating cancer (Kaiser, 2008; Zebrack, 2000). Relative to these understandings, survivors diagnosed at stages I or II and those whose disease has not recurred feel inadequate to claim the survivor label; they feel guilty for having a relatively easy fight with the disease, believing they should have "suffered more." This guilty feeling can undermine women's personal efforts in the survivorship process. Thus, it is refreshing that all survivors do not subscribe to the guilty feeling mentality. Ruth succinctly warns that the cancer experience "is not a competition; there is no winner." She said, "I have heard women tell other women that stage I is not cancer, that stages III and IV are the real ones. You cannot tell somebody that. I always tell them, 'ladies, you cannot out-cancer somebody.' You want to tell me that you getting cancer was any less devastating at stage IV than at stage I? That your stomach did not hit the floor and your jaw dropped? No, you cannot do that."

This concept of survivor's guilt is revealing and offers significant contribution to scholarship on ovarian cancer and cancer survivorship. It suggests that fellow survivors become points of comparison for women; a comparison based on the not-too-pleasant social constructions of the disease. Because of expectations that cancer treatments should be tough in order to be considered effective (Bell, 2009), women go into treatments expecting it to be harsh and difficult. When they construe their experiences as less than the supposed ideal, it produces guilt. Also, it highlights how normative constructions of ovarian cancer and of a cancer survivor become frameworks survivors employ to interpret their lived experiences.

With medical advancements and increasing rates of survival (Markman & Malviya, 2008), survivor's guilt is a reality many ovarian cancer survivors will continue to grapple with. It is, therefore, important to recognize the potential impact of the concept in order to design intervention and support for affected women. Education about survivor's guilt could be incorporated into public education and awareness events; this will help raise awareness and provide caregivers and others the tools to assist survivors. Further, survivor's guilt could be addressed at ovarian cancer support group meetings to ease discomfort in communicating about the issue and open avenues for support seeking and provision. Creating spaces for women to embrace and voice alternative experiences and narratives about the disease would help deconstruct survivor's guilt as a negative aftereffect of the disease. While issues with recurrences may be out of their control, survivors who did not experience recurrences do not have to penalize themselves for their conditions. It is important for scholars, practitioners, and advocates to continue to remind survivors of the factors that contribute to shape the ovarian cancer experience for each woman. This will help curb the practice of comparing experiences among survivors and maximize the potential of support groups and public events as sites of support.

This book argues that women who condone "survivor's guilt" are unknowingly reinforcing beliefs about the disease (e.g., that some cancer experiences are worth more than others, and that ovarian cancer should be tough for it to be real); beliefs they should be challenging because their own experiences contradict these. Women undermine their own experiences to make true erroneous conventional beliefs. I argue that women need an expanded framework to understand and communicatively embody their experiences because frameworks enabled by popular constructions of ovarian cancer and of a cancer survivor are narrow. These frameworks fail to consider effects of diagnosis and treatments on the totality of women's lives. By this, they have encouraged women to unwittingly embrace a survivor-blaming mentality instead of a victor/survivor identity, making it seem uncustomary to survive ovarian cancer.

I argue strongly that women who experience guilt for surviving ovarian cancer have alternative narratives about the disease to offer. These narratives are not in the mainstream; but are needed nonetheless. We need these alternative narratives to help demystify the disease and give an accurate-as-possible representation of the varied experiences on the survivorship continuum. This calls for efforts to increase public education and awareness to help correct the erroneous perceptions. Research and social support efforts are also needed to encourage women to celebrate their individual survival stories; women who feel guilty need to be supported and encouraged to voice, write, and live these alternative narratives. Herein lies the significance of this book which helps put human faces on ovarian cancer and supports alternative narratives and experiences of the disease.

THE SURVIVORSHIP PROCESS

The preceding discussion explains the *process* of ovarian cancer survivorship focusing on the end of active treatments and factors that influence survivors' meaning making processes. The process is illustrated in figure 4.1.

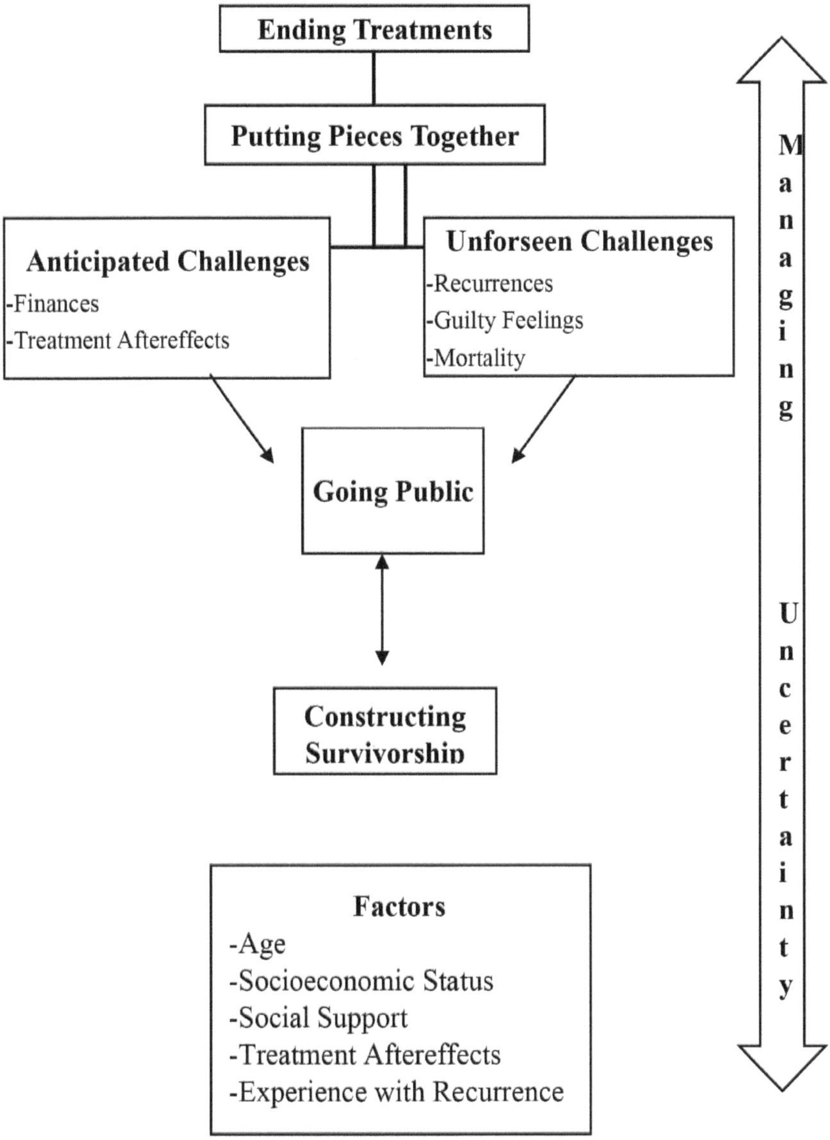

Figure 4.1. The Process of Ovarian Cancer Survivorship

The period following the end of active treatment presents increased uncertainty emanating from experiences with diagnosis and treatments. Uncertainty is high at diagnosis, plateaus during treatments as women focus on actively battling the disease, heightens at the end of treatment, and remains in the backgrounds of women's lives as they navigate treatment aftereffects and/or recurrences. There are no books or explicit rules guiding the path to survivorship, but there are women willing to write and narrate their own lived realities. Women construe their experiences through layered influences of normative views about ovarian cancer and of a cancer survivor, financial stresses, guilt, pride, and social support, which they learn to constructively manage. Complexities and pervasiveness of uncertainty in the illness context (Brashers, 2001) and nature of ovarian cancer point to uncertainty management as integral to the survivorship process. Uncertainty management in the ovarian cancer context is not a one-time occurrence or practice; rather, it is perpetual and integrated into the overall illness experience, especially as chances of disease recurrence increase. Depending on whether women appraise[4] uncertainties as a threat (e.g., uncertainty about one's mortality as a result of deaths in support groups), an opportunity (e.g., uncertainty about disease nature leading to dietary changes and physical exercise), or a chronic situation (e.g., uncertainty about health status and financial security due to severe treatment aftereffects), they use varied communication behaviors to manage these uncertainties. Uncertainties appraised as threats are managed by regulating information and social interaction to decrease or maintain uncertainties (Brashers, 2001). For instance, women who are uncertain about legitimacy of their cancer experiences because of non-recurrences or early diagnoses manage this uncertainty by self-censoring or regulating involvement in support groups. Similarly, women who are uncertain about their mortality and health statuses as a result of deaths in support groups may refrain from joining support groups. And, when women appraise uncertainties as a chronic issue, they accept and adapt to uncertainties. For instance, some women respond to uncertainties about unpredictable health status by choosing to live and plan for the present instead of the distant future. Alternatively, women may frame uncertainties about disease and health as opportunities to adopt healthy lifestyles, including making dietary changes and engaging in physical exercise. As explained previously, women's appraisals of uncertainties and communicative responses, to some extent, are influenced by availability of social and financial resources.

Further, the process of survivorship is unending for some survivors. For women whose disease has recurred, they have yet finished getting back to "normal life" when they have to begin treatment again. The process is not linear as women experience post-treatment issues concurrently.

NOTES

1. Babrow (2001) prefers "coping with" uncertainty to "managing" uncertainty because the latter connotes control over uncertainty, which he believes is impossible. I use "managing uncertainty" in this book to emphasize the agency survivors exercise over their experiences.

2. Some women choose to work during treatments because it helps them maintain a sense of normalcy.

3. Recent research suggests that high prevalence and visibility of breast cancer (as a result of huge survivor support and medical/scientific advances; Koczwara & Ward, 2014) have made breast cancer survivorship the model for all cancer survivorship, including ovarian cancer (Bell, 2014).

4. Appraisal of uncertainties and associated emotional responses are not static (Brashers, 2001). For example, uncertainty appraised as a threat can also be perceived as chronic uncertainty.

Chapter Five

"I Feel Different"

Ovarian Cancer and Sexual Self-Concept[1]

In her op-ed in *The New York Times* in 2013 Angelina Jolie explained she had breast reconstruction surgery following her preventative double mastectomy and noted "It is reassuring that [my children] see nothing that makes them uncomfortable. They can see my small scars and that's it. Everything else is just Mommy, the same as she always was" (Jolie, 2013, para. 12). In an effort to reassure herself and her children that preventative cancer treatments had not changed her, Jolie reified narratives about possible damage cancer treatments can have on the female body, the supposed power reconstructive surgery wields to mask the damage, and perceptions about feminine beauty. Reconstructive surgery presumably can lessen threats of breast cancer to well-being, femininity and the public, and is promoted to women by the medical and cosmetic communities as part of cancer treatment plans (although many women claim the procedure does not meet expectations about mitigating effects of breast loss on sense of worth; Kasper, 1995). As seen in Jolie's case, discussing reconstructive surgery in light of breast cancer presumably makes the disease and treatments less threatening to the public and relational others; there were no apparent deformities or scars on Jolie and her femininity appeared to be intact.[2] However, unlike the breasts, the ovaries (and fallopian tubes) cannot be reconstructed when removed and removal of the ovaries (through a procedure called oophorectomy) can have direr consequences, including menopause, which the public is averse to (Martin, 2001; Ussher, 1989, 2006). Because of associations among women's bodies, positions of specific parts (e.g., breasts and ovaries) on the female body, and notions of femininity and womanhood, effects of cancer treatments on women's sexual self-concept can be debilitating.

In this chapter I extend discussions of ovarian cancer survivorship by analyzing women's interpretations of physical and psychological consequences of treatments on sexual self-concept.[3] I focus on female organs associated with ovarian cancer (i.e., ovary and fallopian tubes) and how perceptions about these organs (including framing of functions of the ovary as defective) shape women's communicative responses to effects of treatments on their sexual self-concept. I discuss factors that influence meanings women construct of their sexual self-concept and highlight how they communicatively manage and negotiate sexual identities and well-being in the face of the life-threatening disease. How do women interpret physical and psychological changes treatments make to their sense of self in light of traditional beauty standards and views about functions of the ovaries? How do women embody these changes in light of the nature of the disease? What roles do women's bodies play in their lived experiences of ovarian cancer? I address these questions below.

EFFECTS OF GYNECOLOGIC CANCER TREATMENTS ON WOMEN

Telling evidences of effects of treatments for gynecologic cancers on women's sexual self-concept include visible and invisible marks on their physical and psychological selves. Scars from surgeries and side effects[4] of treatments, including nausea, tiredness, and neuropathy, provide reminders about changes taking place in women's physical bodies. Side effects of cancer treatments can be more debilitating than the disease itself (Ferrell, Smith, Cullinane & Melancon, 2003) and can put sufferers into a category of the disabled (Ellingson, 2004). Side effects are undeniable (they are felt, seen, and embodied by women) and contribute to some of the psychological changes women experience. Physical effects of gynecologic cancer treatments may recede with time but psychological effects can persist and impact women's self-esteem and relationships (Stead et al., 2001). The intermingling consequences of physical and psychological effects of treatments on women's sexual self-concept are compounded by the extent to which these inhibit women's ability to perform social tasks (i.e., physically caring for children, performing house chores), roles integral to their sense of self (i.e., ability to biologically conceive), and the lenses through which they interpret these effects (e.g., age, treatment protocol, conventional notions about the feminine body).

Changes gynecologic cancer treatments make to women's selves may cause them to feel "different," "insecure," and "traumatized" as they struggle to reconcile current conditions of their physical bodies with the pre-cancer body and perceptions about what a "normal" female body should be, do, and look like. Comparing the pre- and post-cancer body leaves survivors in a state of "dys-embodiment" where the post-cancer body is experienced as dysfunctional and sub-standard to the socially acceptable body (Parton, Ussher & Perz, 2016, p. 494). Research by Parton and colleagues suggests that many female cancer survivors struggle to accept their post-cancer bodies because their post-cancer bodily experiences fall outside the realm of socially sanctioned normality (Parton, Ussher & Perz, 2016). Thus, effects of treatments can disconnect women from their bodies and necessitate they re-learn to accept and understand their bodies (Sekse et al., 2013). For instance, Patricia (67 years, stage III) observed, "When I was in treatment, I was insecure. I felt like a fish out of water; I felt very vulnerable. I really was not myself." Patricia was living in an unknown body and in a foreign space (i.e., hospital), a situation compounded by the intrusion of her body by foreign objects and devices (e.g., medical treatment devices). These events reinforced treatment-related changes she was experiencing in her physical body. The transition from a healthy person to a person socially categorized as sick was quick and evident physically; but Patricia had yet to make the psychological transition. This book, thus, suggests a critical focus on the confluence of physical and psychological location and/or dislocation as important contributors to women's interpretations of effects of treatments on their sexual self-concept.

Similarly, the social and cultural environments in which women inhabit are significant influences in the transformation of physical effects of treatments into psychological scars and wounds. Social factors, including traditional views about the female body, intersect with contextual and demographic variables to impact women's perceptions of effects of treatments on their sexual self-concept. Gynecologic cancers affect organs indicative of womanhood and femininity, such as the ovary, uterus, fallopian tubes, and cervix (Parton, Ussher & Perz, 2015; Sekse et al., 2013; McCallum et al., 2012; Gilbert, Ussher & Perz, 2011; Wilmoth & Spinelli, 2000; Price, 1998). The ovary, for example, holds both medical mystery and dread: it is highly misunderstood and dreaded by the medical community as attempts to understand and tame it have yielded little success (Barker-Benfield, 1972). The ovary is portrayed as a symbol of production and/or non-production, excess, deficiency, monstrosity, and invisibility (Holmes, 2006; Langellier & Sullivan, 1998; Martin, 2001; Stacey, 1997) and as an organ to be wary about (Martin, 1991). And, functions of the ovary (e.g., menstruation and menopause) are considered abnormal (Martin, 2001; Ussher, 1989, 2006). These views about the ovary, in addition to position of the organ in the interior of the female body, contribute to the seeming invisibility of ovarian cancer (Holmes, 2006). However, the ovary is also valued for its reproductive functions (Happe, 2006) and considered an organ essential to womanhood as without it a woman cannot biogenetically conceive. Given the conflicting social and cultural values accorded the ovary and other female organs affected by gynecologic cancers, it is no doubt that effects of treatments for these cancers, including hair loss and changes in structures and functioning of sexual organs, devastate women and present a "sense of injured femininity" (Ferrell, Smith, Cullinane & Melancon, 2003, p. 253). Effects of treatments challenge women's individual and social identities (Hallowell & Lawton, 2002; Krychman & Millheiser, 2013; McCallum et al., 2012; Gilbert, Ussher & Perz, 2011; Vaz et al., 2007; Schultz & van de Wiel, 2003). Parton and colleagues (2015) note that women's perceptions of their post-cancer bodies are impacted by cultural contexts and normative notions about embodied femininity and sexuality. Extending this argument, this book suggests that women's communicative responses to and embodiments of effects of gynecologic cancer treatments are influenced by demographic and contextual factors and also by normative views about the female body and its reproductive functions. The confluence of these impacts needs critical assessment to better appreciate women's embodiments of effects of treatments.

EXPLAINING CONTEXTUAL AND DEMOGRAPHIC FACTORS

Disease-specific, contextual, and demographic factors help explain differences in women's responses to effects of ovarian cancer treatments on their sexual self-concept. Women who are diagnosed at early stages (i.e., stage I or II) and have surgery but not chemotherapy embody effects of treatments differently than those diagnosed at late stages and have combinations of surgery, chemotherapy or radiation treatments. Pre-menopausal women in the former category will not experience induced menopause and associated side effects of hot flashes and hair loss; thus, there may be minimal visible marks of treatments on their bodies. Even though scars from surgeries are present, these may not be visible for public scrutiny; hence, may have minimal impacts on women's sense of self. The less visible marks/effects of treatments are, the lesser their impacts on women's sense of sexual self-concept. For instance, Ann (65 years, stage I), who had surgery but not chemotherapy, noted "[treatment] did not change anything. I look the same, I feel the same." Perhaps the context of Ann's life at the time of her diagnosis and treatment contributed to how she interpreted effects of surgery on her sexual self-concept. Ann's brother died of cancer prior to her diagnosis and her best friend died of cancer shortly after Ann's diagnosis with ovarian cancer. She had these two cancer cases as frames of reference for understanding her own experience. Also, with awareness that ovarian cancer is usually diagnosed at late stages, Ann considered herself lucky her cancer was found early. These events somehow softened Ann's interpretation of effects of treatment on her sexual self-concept. Surviving ovarian cancer helps women to prioritize what is important in life and what is not; many women "changed or downgraded the meaning of sexuality after their illness" (Stewart et al., 2001, p. 541).

On the other hand, however, women diagnosed at late stages (i.e., stages III or IV) have more stringent perceptions of impacts of treatments on their sexual self-concept. Treatments for advanced ovarian cancer, including combinations of surgery and chemotherapy, can leave lasting physical and psychological effects on women (Andersen, 2009; Anderson & Johnson, 1994; Gilbert, Ussher, & Perz, 2010a; Krychman & Millheiser, 2013; Parton, Ussher, & Perz, 2015). When these effects are obvious not only to women but also to society, they can affect women's conceptions of sexual self-concept. For instance, Ruth (55 years old), who was diagnosed with stage IV ovarian cancer and also had preventative double mastectomy, described effects of multiple treatments on her sexual self-concept as follows: "[Treatments] affected the way I perceive myself. I feel so deformed and so ugly; I hate looking at my body in the mirror. I have no interest in having a relationship with a man. I would love to get married but I do not see it in my future. If I cannot stand to look at myself in the mirror, I cannot even imagine a man would." Multiple treatments left both physical and psychological marks on Ruth's life visible not only to herself but also to the public. Inhabiting social spaces where appearance and physicality are privileged (Holmes, 2006), survivors inadvertently interpret their sense of self according to normative standards, which define women and their bodies as inadequate and defective. These expectations add to the stresses women experience adjusting to (and loving) their post-treatment bodies. For example, Ellen (42 years, stage I) explained, "I had 25 staples on my stomach; I came home with drainage tubes because I was still draining. I have scars from my belly all the way down and scars from drainage; so anytime someone made a motion around their stomach I feel that it is because my stomach is fat." Ellen had internalized feminine beauty ideals, which became the framework for surveilling her post-treatment body and interpreting actions of relational others.

Similarly, younger women appear very concerned about permanent marks treatments can leave on their physical and psychological selves, including inability to have children if the ovaries are removed. Losing one's ovaries at an early age will inhibit estrogen production and consequently impact ability to biogenetically conceive. Given general perceptions about fertility and woman's identity (Hallowell & Lawton, 2002), infertility as a result of cancer treatments can be doubly tragic. Treatment-induced infertility can be distressing to younger (ovarian) cancer survivors such that it is considered more traumatic than initial diagnosis (Ferrell, Smith, Cullinane & Melancon, 2003; Ferrell, Smith, Juarez & Melancon, 2003; Yee et al., 2012; Sun, Ramirez & Bodurka, 2007). For instance, Grace (26 years, stage I) explained her reaction to being mistakenly informed hysterectomy had been performed on her. She said, “The nurses were there and I said, ‘Did they do a hysterectomy?’ and both of them looked at me with this terrified look and said ‘yes, they did.’ I could not stop crying for over an hour. Even though I had someone come in [later] to tell me that it did not happen, it was still like the end of the world for me because I want to have a lot of kids.” Research suggests that some women at risk of ovarian cancer appeal to perceptions about reproductive functions of the ovaries to explain why removing these organs negatively impact their sexual self-concept. To these women, the ovaries have “a very material role to play in the maintenance of one’s femininity” (Hallowell & Lawton, 2002, p. 432).

To lessen the “loss” and devastation of cancer treatment-induced infertility, assisted reproductive technologies (ARTs) have become an appealing alternative. ARTs presumably carry promise of possible future genetic pregnancy for cancer survivors (Lockwood, 2002), becoming the “embodied sacrifice” survivors must make to meet normative expectations of motherhood (Martin, 2010, p. 534). The possibility of biologically conceiving through ARTs can be therapeutic and give a sense of hope and control to cancer survivors (Yee et al., 2012). Fertility-preserving options available to cancer survivors include fertility-sparing surgery[5] and embryo, oocyte, or ovarian tissue cryopreservation (i.e., egg freezing). However, distress upon a cancer diagnosis, time constraints (e.g., embryo cryopreservation may require delay in postoperative treatment), lack of adequate information, and cost can limit opportunities for cancer survivors to explore these options (Lee et al., 2006; Yee et al., 2012). As stated previously, ovarian cancer is often diagnosed late, shortening the time between diagnosis and onset of treatment and thus, opportunities to explore fertility preservation options. The urgency to begin treatment can hinder adequate discussion of fertility preservation options between survivors and physicians (Peddie et al., 2012). Taking a critical look at fertility preservation (i.e., egg freezing) for nonmedical reasons, feminist scholars have problematized notions that the procedure empowers women, arguing it puts additional strain on women’s finances and the so-called reproductive autonomy the procedure offers is elusive to many women (Cattapan, Hammond, Haw & Tarasoff, 2014). For instance, many women pay for embryo cryopreservation out of pocket as most insurance plans do not cover assisted reproductive techniques (Lee et al., 2006).

Conversely, older women may not consider consequences of treatments (i.e., removal of ovaries and fallopian tubes) a serious impact on their sexual self-concept. This is because of connections between these organs and reproduction and limited attachment post-menopausal women supposedly have with their reproductive organs. The general perception is that ovaries are of little value aside from their reproductive functions. This means that women who had hysterectomies prior to being diagnosed with ovarian cancer will feel less strongly about effects of treatments on their sexual self-concept.

Although feminist and communication scholars have challenged this view about the ovaries and womanhood (Happe, 2013, 2017), it is still the dominant framework available for women to interpret embodiments of treatment effects.

Women's internalizations of normative views about the ovary manifest in communicative responses to treatments that affect this organ. For instance, Ann (65 years, stage I) stated that "I did not mourn my ovaries and I think it is because I was done with what I needed to do with them; I would have felt a lot different if I still needed to have children. If you no longer need something, you are not going to mourn it if they get taken away." And Carrie (84 years, stage IV) explained, "the doctor suggested I get complete hysterectomy and I said 'fine! I am not using that stuff [i.e., ovaries] anyway and I do not intend to use it again so take it away.'" It is evident Ann and Carrie both had internalized dominant views about their bodies as women, including notions about which body parts are essential to femininity and which are expendable, and appealed to this knowledge to make sense of their experiences. While it may appear this was their own meaning making processes, it is important to understand this meaning making through the lens of societal influences. Women constantly interact with culture that defines the female body and its parts as substandard. Thus, traditional views about reproductive functions of the ovary can negatively and positively impact women's interpretations of effects of treatments on their sexual self-concept.

CHALLENGING NORMATIVE BEAUTY STANDARDS

Western cultural ideals of feminine beauty include views about appeals of the female body to the male sexual gaze, notions about the ideal female body being slender, young, and white, and suggestions to correct imperfections in women (Rubin, Nemeroff & Russo, 2004). In pursuit of these beauty ideals, the female body is disciplined (through practices such as dieting, exercise, makeup use, and cosmetic surgery) but is never successful in attaining these imbalanced, unstable, and unattainable standards (Bartky, 1990). The popular understanding is that mastery of feminine ideals can promote "a secure sense of identity" in women while lack of mastery produces guilt and shame (Bartky, 1990, p. 77). As efforts by women to master these beauty ideals are trivialized by society (i.e., women who pursue these ideals are considered shallow and self-centered), it becomes clear that society's aim is not to help women but subjugate them and point out deficiencies in their bodies (Bartky, 1990). Indeed, our culture teaches women to be insecure bodies and also to see insecure bodies (Bordo, 1993); sexual objectification of the female body is pervasive in Western cultures (Fredrickson & Roberts, 1997). Even though all women (and men) are exposed to, in varying degrees, images and ideologies of feminine beauty, these do not affect all of them equally. Individual life circumstances, including religion, genetics, age, and socio-economic status contribute to how each women is affected by cultural influences (Bordo, 1993; Fredrickson & Roberts, 1997). Internalizing societal beauty ideals leads to self-surveillance in women, self-objectification, feelings of lack and insufficiency, objectification of other women, and some psychological problems (Bartky, 1990; Bordo, 1993; Fredrickson & Roberts, 1997; Rubin, Nemeroff & Russo, 2004). This is because society ties women's social and economic successes to their physical appearance (Fredrickson & Roberts, 1997).

Of course women (and others) resist practices that subordinate women by celebrating diverse female body sizes, shapes, colors, and abilities, challenging normative beauty standards, and through critical consciousness of oppressive systems (Bartky, 1990; Rubin, Nemeroff & Russo, 2004). However, though women are aware and resist practices and discourses that subordinate women, they are limited in the extent to which this knowledge (what Rubin et al., 2004, term "rational resistance") prohibits feelings of self-objectification. This is partly because social structures and systems which objectify women and their lived experiences are the same spaces/channels women must use (and live in) to resist oppressive, normative beauty standards. It is also because, as Susan Bordo (1993) argues,

> Feminist cultural criticism is not a blueprint for the conduct of personal life and does not empower (or require) individuals to "rise above" their culture or to become martyrs to feminist ideals. . . . Its goal is edification and understanding, enhanced *consciousness* of the power, complexity, and *systemic* nature of culture, the interconnected webs of its functioning. It is up to the [individual] to decide how, when, and where (or whether) to put that understanding to further use, in the particular, complicated, and ever-changing context that is his or her life and no one else's (p. 30, emphasis in original).

Pervasiveness of expectations to conform to traditional standards of beauty is undeniable and can affect not only women's sense of self and worth but also their health (Ellingson, 2004). This burden is great in the cancer context where women are simultaneously aware of expectations of the ideal feminine body and limitations placed on their bodies by cancer treatments. In this sense, when faced with choosing cancer treatments, women's concerns rest with choosing treatments that will prolong survival and also treatments that will have minimal effects on their bodies; they are faced with "twin issues of survival and cosmesis" (Kasper, 1995, p. 209). The values society places on the female body and roles certain body parts play in determining femininity and self-esteem influence how women embody cancer and treatments that result in loss of body parts (Kasper, 1995). Cancer survivors whose bodies have been damaged by treatments experience a continuous struggle with "the identity and consequences of being sick in a culture that glorifies health and physical perfection" (Ellingson, 2004, p. 82). For instance, women who have lost a breast to cancer consider the loss devastating to their identities relative to the high social value placed on the female breast (Kasper, 1995). Kasper's (1995) research suggests that women's interpretations of impacts of breast loss on their identities are influenced by socially constructed views about femininity and the female body.

Given dominant societal ideals of beauty against which women must measure their post-cancer-treatment bodies, some ovarian cancer survivors use disciplinary practices Bartky (1990) describes (including wearing scarves, wigs, and makeup) to mask the marks of treatments. Survivors use these items as self-protective mechanisms and also to protect relational others. They want to make their post-treatment bodies less threatening to others and to enhance their own sense of self. For example, Andrea (43 years, stage III) noted she made conscious efforts to present her body in a nonthreatening manner to her children in a bid to make life as normal as possible for them. She said, "It was really important for me to take care of myself because I did not want my children to see me sick. So I never allowed it. I made sure that I got up every day and took a shower and put make-up on. It was hard but I did it." Stella (63 years, stage II) also explained that she covered her head whenever she went into the community so people would not be offended by her bald head: "I would sit on the front porch with my bald head and it did not bother me. But I would wear a hat to the store simply because I did not want to offend anybody that might see me with a bald head and not like it."

The burden on women to adjust their post-treatments bodies to meet societal standards of "normal," "feminine," and "healthy" can be debilitating and can limit women's efforts to fully embody their experiences. This can impact women's conceptions of their sexual self-concept, add a layer of stress to their experiences of the disease, and highlight challenges of living in and communicating about effects of a hard-to-visualize disease (Holmes, 2006). Feminist scholars (e.g., Butler & Rosenblum, 2001; Lorde, 1997) argue societal standards and demands of beauty rob women of the agency to embody their lived experiences. How society reacts to women who have no hair compels affected women to constantly explain their health status; women who want to avoid giving explanations and to feel normal, choose to cover their scars and head. The desire to feel "normal" post-cancer explains why most women choose to have breast reconstruction following treatments for breast cancer (Rubin & Tanenbaum, 2011). With ovarian cancer, the quest for normalcy causes women to magnify the insidiousness of, say, hysterectomy or oophorectomy.

TRANSCENDING PHYSICAL SCARS: ROLE OF RELATIONAL OTHERS IN WOMEN'S RESPONSES TO SEXUAL AND EMBODIED CHANGES AFTER CANCER

Support from social networks is crucial as women negotiate effects of cancer treatments on perceptions about sexual self-concept. Although women may not always and/or directly solicit it, support can prove vital to their meaning making processes. This is because changes in women's bodies are communicated and embodied through interpersonal interactions with others in their social environments and because relational partners (much as survivors) are affected by cancer and its treatments. Because of the interdependent nature of (romantic) relationships, both patients and their partners are impacted by illness experiences (Coyne & Smith, 1991; Goldsmith, 2009). For instance, many partners of individuals treated for cancer have expressed how the cancer experience affected their sexual relationships with survivors. Issues such as treatment side effects (e.g., fatigue and loss of sexual desire) and consequences of the caring role (which repositions the person with cancer as a patient instead of a partner) can impact sexual relationships between partners (Gilbert, Ussher & Perz, 2010; Hawkins et al., 2009). Survivors, particularly women, care about whether their partners find their post-cancer-treatment bodies attractive (see Miller & Coughlin, 2013). Thus, the way partners respond to changes treatments make to survivors' bodies can help reinforce or ameliorate the distress survivors experience in relation to the embodied changes.

Research suggests that romantic partners differ in their coping strategies and how openly they communicate about illness-related distress. While some of them consider the illness experience a relational issue with implications for both partners, others appraise and communicate about the illness experience and its effects as an individual issue—approaches scholars term "active engagement" and "protective buffering," respectively (Coyne & Smith, 1991) or "mutual responsiveness" and "disengaged avoidance" (Kayser, Watson & Andrade, 2007). Approaching the illness experience as a relational issue helps couples to communicate openly about their stresses and identify ways to support each other; it also enables couples to renegotiate intimacy and sexuality during and/or after a cancer experience. Renegotiating intimacy and sexuality includes couples finding other means besides penetrative intercourse to be sexually intimate (Gilbert et al., 2010). On the contrary, considering the cancer experience as an individual issue inhibits communication and support provision (Kayser et al., 2007), among other issues. Communication and positive relational context play important roles in how couples renegotiate sexual issues during a cancer experience (Gilbert et al., 2010).

Thus, support and affirmation from partners, family members, friends, coworkers, and support group members can be instrumental in helping ovarian cancer survivors move past the physical and psychological scars and limitations imposed by treatments. Available social support can significantly ameliorate effects of treatments on sexual self-concept regardless of contextual and demographic factors. Younger and older women diagnosed at different stages of the disease may appraise effects of treatment on their sexual self-concept differently. But the support each woman receives can help put these changes into perspective and determine the level of significance these take in her life. For instance, Mercy (58 years, stage I) explained how being part of a cancer workout support group helped her regain her self-confidence after treatment. She noted, "[The support group] helped me gain my self-confidence back because with my chemo, no matter what I did I gained 10–15 pounds; and I just did not look like myself. I had no hair, I had no eyelashes, I had no eyebrows." Andrea also mentioned how support she received from family and friends helped her take pride in the physical scars from treatments.

However, lack of support from society and relational others can hamper efforts women make to incorporate effects of treatment into their sexual self-concept. Lack of support include instances when others question legitimacy of women's experiences because women do not "look" like a cancer patient (i.e., weak and without hair) or when others react negatively to effects of treatments on women. For instance, Ellen (42 years, stage I) explained people questioned if she had cancer because she only had surgery but not chemotherapy. She said, "My mother-in-law once made the comment that 'well, you didn't really have cancer' and I'm like I don't get what that mean. And she said, 'you didn't do chemo and radiation.'" To Ellen's mother-in-law, chemotherapy and radiation treatments were the seal of legitimacy of a cancer experience, therefore, any cancer experience devoid of these treatments was not *really* cancer. In instances as Ellen's, women leave the responsibility to appreciate their cancer experiences to others to figure out, realizing limits to their efforts to make treatment effects meaningful and less threatening to others. To many women, changes in their post-treatment bodies are the evidences society needs to see to start rethinking conventional views of the "healthy," "feminine," and "normal" body because these standards lose substance in the ovarian cancer context. For instance, Patricia (67 years, stage III) explained how having no hair made her cancer experience real to her brother who stared at her for the entire period he visited. She stated, "My brother had a hard time sitting there looking at me with no hair because that made [my cancer] very real to him. I could see it all over his face; he just kept looking at me and his lips quivered because with the hair gone, it made it real to him." For Patricia, the changes in her physical body were part of her ovarian cancer experience; she did not need to change anything about that.

Rather, the onus rested with those who could not accept the "difference" in her body to learn to appreciate it as presented to them; those people needed to acknowledge that following treatment for ovarian cancer, women's strength is connected with looking different and weak, contrary to popular standards.

This book argues that it is not only how ovarian cancer survivors see themselves with physical and psychological scars from treatments that impact their conceptions of sexual self-concept. Rather, how relational others and society respond to differences treatments make to women's bodies is implicative for women's conceptions about effects of treatments. Women's bald heads and surgery-induced scars automatically communicate to society that women are different—a difference that challenges normative standards of beauty. Indeed, effects of cancer treatments on sexuality and sexual health depends on personal characteristics as well as social and contextual factors (Schultz & van de Wiel, 2003; Price, 1995). Similarly, in the case of ovarian cancer, physical effects of treatments alone do not affect women's understandings of sexual self-concept; instead, their perceptions are shaped by contextual and demographic factors and normative views about the feminine body. The damage of ovarian cancer treatments on women's physical and psychological selves has the potential to negatively impact their perceptions of sexual self-concept. However, whether these changes take center stage in women's embodiments of their experiences is moderated by other external factors.

In the case of ovarian cancer, it is in the image of a sick, scarred, and worn-out body that women are sure they are well or are getting rid of the disease. It is when women look sick with no hair, that they are assured they are actually well and healthy. This draws partly from cultural meanings of suffering (that it should be purposeful) which infiltrates cancer survivors' perceptions of treatments (Bell, 2009). But, it is also because the disease may be lurking in women's bodies without them knowing given its insidious nature; thus, the physical side effects of treatments provide visible evidence and reminders that treatments are effective. In this context, then, the end of treatments, which would normally be hailed because women's bodies get to rejuvenate, presents uncertainty and anxiety to ovarian cancer survivors because they can no longer trust the "normal" body and the social environment in which it inhabits. Looking ahead, it is imperative to ask: How should these factors/issues shape advocacy around the disease and efforts to encourage survivors to take control over their experiences? How might women's conceptions of survivorship and interpretations of effects of treatments on their sense of self manifest in the practice of self-advocacy? How do characteristics of ovarian cancer (e.g., late diagnosis, recurrences, and permanent effects of treatments) challenge popular conceptions of self-advocacy in the cancer context? I explore these questions in the next chapter.

NOTES

1. An earlier version of this chapter was published by Taylor & Francis Group in *Women's Reproductive Health* on 21 March, 2017, available online: http://dx.doi.org/10.1080/23293691.2017.1276371. (Tetteh, D. (2017). "I feel different": Ovarian cancer and sexual self-concept. *Women's Reproductive Health* [Special issue on Cancer and Women's Reproductive Health], 4(1), 61-73.)

2. Research suggests Jolie's sexuality was frequently referenced in discourses around her medical announcements (Dean, 2016).

3. Sexual self-concept is a component of sexual health. Sexual health comprises *sexual function* (including desire, arousal/excitement, and orgasm), *sexual self-concept* (including body image, sexual esteem, and sexual self-schema), and *sexual roles and relationships* (including communication and intimacy) (Cleary & Hegarty, 2011; Woods, 1987).

4. Treatment side effects can be temporary or permanent and can affect survivors' physical and psychological health. See Sun, Ramirez & Bodurka (2007) for discussions about these impacts on survivors' quality of life.

5. The type of surgery depends on ovarian tumor type (i.e., epithelial, borderline, or germ cell) and stage of diagnosis (i.e., late or early stage) (Feichtinger & Rodriguez-Wallberg, 2016).

Chapter Six

Advocacy and Self-Advocacy in the Ovarian Cancer Context

With Gini Steinke, founder and executive director of Ovarian Cancer Connection, Toledo, Ohio

A 2013 study published in the *Journal of Advanced Nursing* sought to define and differentiate self-advocacy in cancer survivorship from related concepts. To that end, the authors, Teresa Hagan and Heidi Donovan, professors in the Department of Acute and Tertiary Care at the University of Pittsburgh School of Nursing, used the cases of two ovarian cancer survivors as "real-world exemplars" to illustrate what was and was not self-advocacy (p. 2350). A thorough search of existing literature helped the researchers design a model of self-advocacy, which comprised attributes of the concept[1] and antecedents (e.g., personal characteristics, learned skills, and attainability of support). Ovarian cancer survivors in the case study were part of a web-based intervention called Written Representational Intervention to Ease Symptoms (WRITE Symptoms). The intervention was designed to help survivors with recurrent ovarian cancer manage symptoms. Survivors interacted with research nurses by describing symptoms they were experiencing via private message boards to which the nurses responded by providing individualized symptom management information to help survivors take control of their symptoms (Ward, Heidrich & Donovan, 2007). The cases of two survivors, Judy and Anne, were presented by Hagan and Donovan to illustrate self-advocacy and a lack of it.

Judy's posts on the WRITE platform were explained as representing self-advocacy in that she possessed characteristics of a self-advocate (e.g., drive to overcome challenges and try new things), she had excellent communication, information-seeking, and problem-solving skills, and was able to access available resources. "In response to her severe and distressing cancer-related symptoms, Judy ends up advocating for herself in a way that gives her a renewed self-concept and hope for the future with a better sense of control over cancer and chemotherapy's symptoms: 'It seems like it has been a long time since I have felt so happy and free'" (Hagan & Donovan, 2013b, p. 2355). On the other hand, Anne's posts were assessed as embodying non-self-advocacy. The authors explained,

> Considering Anne's lack of antecedents to self-advocacy, her difficulty in self-advocating is not surprising. Instead of creating a 'new normal,' taking ownership of her cancer and feeling empowered, her thoughts and cognitions seem stuck in feeling victimized by the cancer and her healthcare team and unable to move out of a state of passivity and regret. She is unable to navigate the healthcare system effectively, make informed choices that benefit her, or build teamwork with her care team. Anne does not mention any availability or use of outside support groups or organizations. She does not indicate having a source of support or encouragement. Without the key attributes of self-advocacy, she continues to struggle with poorly managed symptoms and feels hopeless and frustrated (Hagan & Donovan, 2013b, p. 2355).

Anne's honest communication about her feelings deviated from the standard cancer narrative of enthusiasm and hope; thus, she was characterized as a non-self-advocate. Missing from Hagan and Donovan's (2013b) analysis was legitimization of Anne's feelings made possible by investigating the cancer experience from her perspective and recognition of differences in cancer survivors' embodiments of control over their experiences.

Following her diagnosis with breast cancer and subsequent mastectomy, prominent feminist scholar Audre Lorde (1997) expressed value in developing her "own internal sense of power" as survival and resistance strategies, noting that women have a "militant responsibility" to be informed about and involved in their own health (p. 75). However, Lorde also argued that a "clear distinction must be made between this affirmation of self and the superficial farce of "looking on the bright side of things" because "looking on the bright side of things is a euphemism used for obscuring certain realities of life, the open consideration of which might prove threatening or dangerous to the status quo" (p. 76). While Lorde supports women's responsibility and right to be involved in their health care, she also cautions against discrediting women's anger and sufferings under the guise of self-advocacy. Thus, a critical analysis of self-advocacy (i.e., one's ability to stand up for him/herself, seek information, and be involved in health care decisions) and advocacy (i.e., defense of oneself, another, or others; Temple, 2002) and looking on the bright side of things in the ovarian cancer context demands we ask: How does labeling certain behaviors as self-advocacy and/or non-self-advocacy work to discredit some cancer experiences and encourage a monolithic perspective about self-advocacy? How does so-called non-self-advocacy threaten the status quo of expected behaviors of women and the ill? How do cancer experiences such as Anne's challenge normative discourses of cancer advocacy and self-advocacy?

There is no denying the exigency of self-advocacy in the ovarian cancer context given the medical community's disregard for women's complaints about symptoms which consequently leads to late diagnosis. Circumstances surrounding diagnosis rob women of their voices such that self-advocacy becomes a realistic means to regain control over their experiences. However, there is a problem with self-advocacy (as commonly promoted in the cancer context) when normative beliefs about the ill and women's bodies and health (which put women in positions of disempowerment and voicelessness in the first place) become the same belief systems from which guidelines about how women should self-advocate are drawn. There is a problem when these normative beliefs are flipped, repackaged, and offered as self-empowering tools to women. Because in essence these so-called models of self-advocacy ask survivors to play by hegemonic rules in order for efforts to claim control over their experiences to be validated and legitimized.

In this chapter, we conceptualize ovarian cancer advocacy and self-advocacy by tracing history of the women's health movement and (breast) cancer advocacy in the United States. Drawing from communication, feminist and critical cultural scholarship, we discuss how widespread promotion of self-advocacy in the cancer context burdens survivors and encourages individual responsibility for health and illness. Specifically, we critique the "think positive" discourse and the guilt and/or blame it inflicts on cancer survivors. A main argument of this book is that while self-advocacy in the cancer context seemingly gives control over their health care to women, understanding the aims, foci, priorities, and sponsors of advocacy organizations/groups can help better explicate how expectations and demands of self-advocacy further hegemonic norms and constrain varied embodiments of control over the cancer experience. We contend that rigid interpretations of self-advocacy serve the interests of corporate sponsors who need evidence (i.e., drastic transformations in women's cancer experiences) to determine value for monetary investments (in the name of philanthropy) made toward cancer advocacy. We use the Ovarian Cancer Connection (OCC) as a case study and draw from its organizing principles to highlight appropriate models of advocacy in the ovarian cancer context. This form of advocacy carries promise of encouraging self-advocacy and self-affirmation in the direst circumstances when survivors, due to health reasons, may not be able to embody normative self-advocacy.

THE OVARIAN CANCER CONNECTION

The OCC is a nonprofit ovarian cancer support organization in Toledo, Ohio, United States. It was founded in 2005 by nine women who were either survivors of ovarian cancer or knew someone diagnosed with the disease. Previously known as National Ovarian Cancer Coalition of NW Ohio and SE Michigan, the OCC severed ties in 2010 with the National Ovarian Cancer Coalition (NOCC) to become an independent nonprofit organization. This decision stemmed from a desire to use all funds raised locally to support survivors in the local area. The OCC is supported by the community and run by an all-volunteer staff; it also partners with local health workers and health institutions to support ovarian cancer survivors and their families. The OCC provides financial[2] and material support (e.g., it pays utility and rent/mortgage bills for survivors and provides transportation to medical appointments) for ovarian cancer (and recently all gynecologic cancer) survivors and also advocates for ovarian cancer research and education. The OCC relies on two major events to raise funds—the Ellen Jackson Ovarian Cancer Walk which takes place in September every year and Tee Off for Teal in Memory of Karen Creque.

CANCER ADVOCACY IN WESTERN SOCIETIES

The changing health care landscape in Western societies has ushered in an era of care where compliance as well as assertiveness are expected of patients. Patients are expected to be knowledgeable about their disease conditions and contribute to treatment decisions. It is believed when patients are involved in treatment decision making it can positively impact health outcomes, empowerment, shared responsibility, respect, and mutual trust between patients and physicians (Andersen et al., 2012; Barry & Edgman-Levitan, 2012; IOM, 2013; Mead et al., 2013; Peek et al. 2013). However, severity of some health conditions, including cancer, makes it difficult for sufferers to meet expectations of the assertive, outspoken, and compliant patient, as some of them may still be recovering from the shock of diagnosis when decisions about treatments need to be made. Many cancer survivors find it overwhelming to navigate complex health care systems, a situation that can compromise ability to make informed decisions and effectively evaluate treatment plans (O'Hair et al., 2003). Given that communication between survivors and health care providers is crucial in cancer care (O'Hair et al., 2003), advocacy efforts (in and outside medical settings) are essential to help center survivors' voices. Considered a process of defending oneself, another, or others (Temple, 2002), advocacy in the cancer context has a long history in the United States, beginning with the women's health movement which is credited for not only championing women's health issues but also helping bring awareness to (breast) cancer as a social issue (Ruzek & Becker, 1999).

To understand advocacy related to specific cancers and women's health in Western societies, it is important to present a history of the women's health movement in the United States in the 1970s and 1980s and how the cancer advocacy landscape evolved into what it is today. (See Doyal (1983) for a discussion of history of the women's health movement in Britain). A detailed history of the women's health movement at the grassroots level and emergence of professional women's health advocacy groups in the United States was provided by Ruzek and Becker (1999). The grassroots women's health movement championed raising consciousness of women, their bodies and health by becoming patient advocates (where activists accompanied individual women to doctor's appointments), providing health-related services to women (e.g., referral, abortion, gynecologic, and obstetric services), and arguing for legitimacy of women's subjective knowledge about their bodies and health (Marieskind, 1975; Ruzek & Becker, 1999). With the aim of empowering women to define their own health experiences, efforts by the grassroots movement encouraged transfer of knowledge about women's health from male experts to women themselves (Ruzek & Becker, 1999). However, the social context and health advocacy landscape changed in the late 1980s as organizers and founders of the women's health movement returned to paid work, started families, or went back to school—changes that reduced available pool of volunteers (Ruzek & Becker, 1999). Indeed, membership of the movement, which comprised women of varied socioeconomic classes, ages and ethnicities, was its "greatest strengths and energy sources" (Marieskind, 1975, p. 220). Not only were there changes in the structure of the grassroots group but there were also changes at the national and state levels with the influx of mainstream health institutions and nonprofit groups in women's health care (Ruzek & Becker, 1999). These professional organizations were well-organized and sponsored by large hospitals and pharmaceutical corporations, which influenced their organizing, foci, and priorities in the services they provided women. For instance, Avon, a global vendor of beauty products and a sponsor of breast cancer awareness programs, founded the Worldwide Fund for Women's Health in 1992 to support initiatives related to women's health[3] (King, 2006). The proliferation and prominence of professional advocacy groups affected operations of grassroots movements as the former received the majority of federal funding and aligned their operations with the aims of corporate sponsors (e.g., prioritizing single women's health issues; Ruzek & Becker, 1999). As part of what is known as "strategic philanthropy," corporations prefer to support specific health issues (e.g., breast cancer) and make donations that align with corporate goals and aims so as to satisfy corporate social responsibility and attract potential customers (King, 2006). This single-issue advocacy strategy attracted professional women who did not necessarily identify as feminist but whose aims aligned with the foci of professional organizations (Ruzek & Becker, 1999).

Breast cancer advocacy groups (e.g., the National Breast Cancer Coalition; NBCC) were among successful disease-specific professional advocacy groups in the United States to form alliances with consumers, medical professionals, researchers, and survivors to bring awareness about the disease and advocate for funding for research and support services (Ruzek & Becker, 1999). The NBCC was successful in attracting federal funding for research related to breast cancer but the majority of this funding and awareness has focused on early detection through mammogram rather than disease prevention and treatments for underserved populations (King, 2006). As Ellen Leopold (1999) explains in her book on the history of breast cancer in America, cancer organizations' concerns with treatments rather than prevention and research instead of equitable access to treatment reflect the interests and perspectives of leaders of these organizations who are mostly affluent, educated, and had ties with the medical establishment. Indeed, in the current for-profit economy, corporate sponsors consider investment in cancer treatments more profitable than investing in prevention efforts (Lorde, 1997). Associations between disease-specific professional advocacy groups and corporate sponsors, their orientation toward social change, attitude toward biomedicine, among others, have implications for how they operate and advocate for women's health (King, 2006; Ruzek & Becker, 1999). Thus, though both the grassroots women's health groups and professional, disease-specific advocacy groups sought to improve women's health care, their foci and priorities varied relative to the aims and for-profit interests of their sponsors. For instance, the breast cancer movement in the United States, spearheaded by organizations such as the National Alliance of Breast Cancer Organizations (NABCO) and the NBCC, lacks feminist and activist orientation partly because of the interests of corporate leaders and sponsors, including pharmaceutical companies (King, 2006). Breast cancer has become an appealing health issue which for-profit corporations (e.g., Avon) use to advance corporate interests, a situation that raises questions about the authenticity of corporate philanthropy supporting women's health issues and breast cancer specifically (King, 2006).

Increased interest in single-issue women's health advocacy relative to requirements for federal funding and attractiveness of single health issues for corporate interests propelled the breast cancer movement and later helped draw national attention to ovarian cancer as a women's health issue (Ruzek & Becker, 1999). Thus, advocacy around ovarian cancer (and other diseases) mirrored[4] that around breast cancer with a high focus on awareness, early detection and individual responsibility for health rather than prevention and a focus on broader issues of inequality and discrimination (see King, 2006).

This narrow approach to cancer advocacy is evident in the work of ovarian cancer advocacy groups such as the National Ovarian Cancer Coalition (NOCC), which promote early detection through awareness. The NOCC aims to educate and increase awareness about ovarian cancer and recognizes that, "There is currently no early detection test for ovarian cancer. . . . Until there is a screening test, the key to early diagnosis is awareness" (NOCC, n.d, para. 2). In April 2017 the NOCC received a $50,000 "Health in Your Hands" grant[5] from Quest Diagnostics, a global provider of diagnostic information services (e.g., genetic tests), to support its programs and services to ovarian cancer survivors and caregivers (Hunt, 2007). It also received a $100,000 donation from Pureology, a subsidiary of the beauty product giant L'Oréal USA in 2017. Pureology would sponsor NOCC's 2017 *Run/Walk to Break Silence on Ovarian Cancer*. The NOCC continues to enjoy support from corporate partners such as Counsy (a DNA testing and genetic counseling service provider), Abcodia (a company that develops tests for early detection of cancer), Mary Kay, and AstraZeneca—support that is fantastic and shows willingness of society to support ovarian cancer-related causes; but it can influence how NOCC operates and advocates for ovarian cancer survivors.

Also worth mentioning are roles played by survivor-led groups such as the National Coalition of Cancer Survivorship (NCCS) in the cancer advocacy movement. The NCCS aims to include the voices of survivors at higher levels of policy and decision-making. The success of the NCCS includes spearheading formation of the Office of Cancer Survivors within the National Cancer Institute (NCI), which subsequently led to increased funding for the NCI and public awareness about cancer survivorship (Bell & Ristovski-Slijepcevic, 2013). The NCI also initiated the Consumer Advocates in Research and Related Activities (CARRA) to liaise between cancer survivors and the NCI (Temple, 2002). Membership of CARRA comprises cancer survivors, people closely related to survivors, or those with experience working with/for cancer survivors (Temple, 2002).

Efforts by these advocacy groups and individual survivors have been effective in impacting policy changes, research, funding, and awareness about cancer, including ovarian cancer (Committee on the State of the Science in Ovarian Cancer Research et al., 2016; Temple, 2002). Members of these organizations have fought for (and gained) voting privileges and participation in funding/grant review and advisory committees in the United States Department of Defense and the Food and Drug Administration, for instance, where they advocate for the rights of cancer survivors (Temple, 2002). Successes of these organizations point to an emerging trend in society where the views and experiences of cancer survivors are increasingly being recognized and incorporated into "the fabric of the cancer establishment" (King, 2006, p. 107). The work of these organizations highlight ways in which cancer survivors have used their own experiences to draw attention to the disease and advocate for women's complaints about symptoms to be taken seriously by the medical community. For instance, women played a crucial role in drawing physicians' attention to signs of early-stage ovarian cancer even as medical textbooks claimed the disease presented no symptoms at early stages (Twombly, 2007).

However, there are problems with how these large organizations approach cancer advocacy. Few of these advocacy groups (e.g., Breast Cancer Action) encourage critical engagements with the medical establishment and voicing anger and frustration against inequalities and discriminations in social structures (King, 2006). While this may be a calculated strategy by advocacy groups to garner support and funding from political, medical, and corporate actors using nonthreatening and aggressive approaches, it has diverted attention away from core societal issues that contribute to the cancer epidemic and has created an erroneous mindset about cancer and survivors (e.g., that cancer is nonthreatening and survivors are heroic and optimistic; King, 2006). These professional advocacy groups are interested in promoting brands rather than realities of the disease (Sulik, 2012). Similar to successes of the women's health movement in increasing public awareness about women's health and influencing related medical research (Dubriwny, 2013), the breast cancer movement has helped demystify the disease and increased public awareness and education. However, it has also led to sexualization of women's bodies, taken attention away from realities of the disease, and alienated women who choose not to embody conceptions of the optimistic, heroic, and brave survivor (Sulik, 2012). This has been a key contention of feminist and critical scholars against professional cancer advocacy organizations. These scholars argue that though professional advocacy groups attempt to speak for women, they do not in that they lack activist and feminist mindsets in their organizing (Hill, 2016; King, 2006; Ruzek & Becker, 1999; Sulik, 2012)

In this context, local nonprofit cancer advocacy groups whose primary aim is to support survivors and encourage self-affirmation become significant players in helping redefine advocacy. These organizations do not only educate about the disease but also stand for and with survivors. For example, the OCC plays a much-needed advocacy role in walking hand-in-hand with women diagnosed with ovarian cancer by providing basic needs often ignored by society and professional advocacy groups. The majority of women the OCC supports are "single women caring for young children. These women have emptied their financial resources and are on the verge of utility disconnection, eviction, and struggling to maintain a healthy diet for their children let alone themselves," according to Gini Steinke, founder and executive director of the OCC. To receive support from the OCC, women must be referred by a medical professional or they can call the OCC office directly.

Leaders of the OCC follow up with a call to women and begin a very private conversation not only about women's recent diagnosis but their financial situations also. Gini explains that "sometimes it can take weeks or months for a survivor to reach out to the OCC because as we all know, it can be very difficult for anyone to ask for help of any kind." She narrates, "In 2016, I received a call from a social worker asking me to call a young woman with two young children under the age of 12 recently diagnosed with stage III ovarian cancer. A proud woman with an excellent job who always had a nest egg for emergencies and in one day her life changed dramatically. When I called her, immediately she began to cry, she shared with me that the gas to heat her home was to be disconnected in five days, she had very little food to feed her children and she just received an eviction notice from her landlord. Her diagnosis immediately threw her into a financial nightmare. Within two days, the OCC paid her gas bill, worked with her landlord to avoid eviction, delivered a $100 gift card from a local grocery store that was donated to the OCC and made a referral to Nightingale Harvest, a local food bank for cancer patients. Over the course of her treatments, the OCC continued to assist her until she was in remission. Should the cancer return, the OCC will be ready to aid again."

Women supported by the OCC are those whose voices are silenced by mainstream advocacy approaches focusing on early detection and fundraising. Indeed, society, including legislators, find it safe, less controversial, and politically beneficial to support awareness and early detection efforts around women's health issues (e.g., breast cancer) than to address failures in the social structure that cause these issues. They also shy away from providing tangible aid to those affected, including expanding medical coverage for sufferers from low-income backgrounds (King, 2006). For instance, many health insurance companies in the United States do not pay for predictive testing and preventative treatments for women at risk of hereditary breast and ovarian cancer (HBOC) even though the Patient Protection and Affordable Care Act (PPACA) mandates coverage for these services (US DHHS, 2010). In many instances, at-risk women have to go through lengthy procedures to appeal non-coverage decisions by their health insurance companies. Further, research suggests ovarian cancer survivors treated by gynecologic oncologists have a better chance of survival than those who are treated by general physicians; however, very few survivors have access to this high-quality care as these specialists are rare and over-burdened (Bristow, Chang, Ziogas, Randall & Anton-Culver, 2014). In the case of breast cancer, a breast cancer research stamp introduced in 1998 to raise funds to support breast cancer research received bilateral support from national legislators whereas very few legislators came on board "When support for the fight against breast cancer takes the form of providing Medicaid coverage for the treatment of low-income women diagnosed with breast and cervical cancer, or providing coverage for the routine patient care costs of Medicare beneficiaries who are participating in clinical trials, or enacting a comprehensive and enforceable Patients' Bill of Rights, or passing law to prohibit public health insurance and employment discrimination based on genetic information" (King, 2006, p. 78)

As argued by Dubriwny (2013), there is no specific way to enact feminist health activism given the changing social and political landscapes and practices of women's health politics. Instead, all health advocacy and/or support groups have opportunities to add activist orientations to the work they do where they do not totally reject the biomedical industry but take a critical stance to its operations and claims (Dubriwny, 2013). Dubriwny (2013) calls for new feminist health politics with an "activist orientation that includes both a recognition of the promise of biomedicine and a recognition of its dangers" (p. 157). This is pertinent because while it may not be practical for all women's health advocacy organizations to reject corporate sponsorship; they can maintain a critical view about biomedical knowledge and broadly conceptualize women's health (Dubriwny, 2013). Dubriwny (2013) cites work by the grassroots breast cancer organization Breast Cancer Action (BCA) to suggest that women's health activist groups need to be educated and abreast of current biomedical knowledge and advances to effectively advocate for women's health. The BCA plays a watchdog role and critically assesses new biomedical advances in breast cancer treatment and opposes those deemed harmful to women (Dubriwny, 2013).

Dubriwny's (2013) argument helps situate the OCC as an advocacy organization. The OCC's organizing principles include valuing every woman's experience and helping her find her voice and strength during diagnosis, treatment, and life afterward. The leaders do not seek any material reward (the organization is run by all volunteers). They go to Capitol Hill each year to advocate for increased funding for ovarian cancer research. The organization also plans to take its advocacy efforts to the classrooms of medical schools through the Survivors Teaching Students program (STS)[6] where ovarian cancer survivors use their lived experiences to teach medical students about the disease and often overlooked symptoms. Because medical students are the future physicians who will be treating and caring for women with gynecologic cancers, survivors are in a unique position to help them become more sensitive to the symptoms of the disease and to show that survival is possible. "STS brings the faces and voices of ovarian cancer survivors into the classrooms of undergraduate medical, nursing, social work, and pharmacy students" (Fitch, McAndrew, Turner, Ross, & Pison, 2011).

SELF-ADVOCACY IN THE CANCER CONTEXT

The cancer survivorship movement in the 1980s spearheaded by survivors and survivor-led groups has helped change perspectives about cancer (e.g., from a death sentence to a survivable disease) and increased awareness about the poignant voices survivors carry in defining their own experiences (Clark & Stovall, 1996). The movement has empowered cancer survivors to stand up for themselves, seek information, and be involved in decisions concerning their health care (i.e., self-advocacy). This is imperative given the changing realm of cancer care (i.e., from an acute illness into a chronic illness), the changing needs of survivors in the survivorship trajectory (e.g., informational and support needs), and the need to center and prioritize survivors' voices in support and intervention initiatives (Clark & Stovall, 1996; Hoffman & Stovall, 2006). Further, emphasis on the patient-centered model as the ideal model of health care has increased expectations of survivors to be actively involved in managing their own disease symptoms and treatment side effects; hence, a need for survivors to be able to self-advocate (Hagan & Donovan, 2013a). Self-advocacy is believed to positively contribute to health outcomes, including patient empowerment and quality of life. Hence, widespread acceptance of the concept in the cancer survivorship context; it has support among practitioners, scholars, and patients (Hagan & Donovan, 2013b).

Cancer survivors need specific set of skills to effectively self-advocate and adapt to the cancer experience. These include skills in communication, information-seeking and processing, self-education about disease and treatment options, problem-solving, negotiation, and assertiveness (Brashers, Haas & Neidig, 1999; Clark & Stovall, 1996; Hagan & Donovan, 2013b; Hoffman & Stovall, 2006; Wright, Frey & Sopory, 2007). Moreover, literacy skills such as reading, numeracy, speaking, and listening are needed to self-advocate (Martin et al., 2011); as well as willingness to communicate about one's health issues with health care providers (Wright, Frey & Sopory, 2007) and the inner drive to overcome or control the cancer experience (Hagan & Donovan, 2013b). Possessing these skills and the extent to which they are exercised can make a difference in the choices survivors make regarding care (e.g., seeking a second opinion, and treatment options) and control they exert over their experiences (O'Hair et al., 2003). For example, with these skills, survivors can navigate complex health care systems, utilize available resources (e.g., social support) and information to make informed, rational decisions about their health (including knowing when to discontinue treatment and adhere to medical recommendation), use their experiences to support and guide others facing similar health problems, and identify with the larger cancer community (Hagan & Donovan, 2013b). Importantly, self-advocacy skills can be developed and nurtured in survivors through training and education (Clark & Stovall, 1996).

The notion that self-advocacy is realized when survivors experience a sense of control over the disease, adjust to life with cancer, and attain a strong self-concept (Hagan & Donovan, 2013b) raises serious concerns about assumptions about self-advocacy. Research points to discrepancies between popular conceptions of self-advocacy and how it is embodied by survivors. Contrary to standard definitions of self-advocacy (as a set of skills survivors need to adapt and make their voices heard during medical encounters), many cancer survivors consider self-advocacy a means to keeping a positive attitude and battling the disease (Hagan & Medberry, 2016). For instance, the National Coalition for Cancer Survivorship (NCCS) considers information seeking one of the skills necessary for cancer survivors to effectively self-advocate; however, some cancer survivors do not consider information seeking one of the ways they self-advocate (Hagan & Medberry, 2016). Indeed, avoiding seeking information is a strategy for managing illness-related uncertainty (Brashers et al., 2009). And, some individuals prefer to leave treatment decisions to physicians (Levinson, Kao, Kuby & Thisted, 2005). These are critical issues often not highlighted in the self-advocacy scholarship.

PROBLEMS WITH SELF-ADVOCACY

Adding their intellectual voices to self-advocacy in the cancer context, feminist and critical/cultural scholars have argued that it is important to define self-advocacy for the purposes of research, but also warned that such categorization can exclude the experiences of survivors who do not embody standard definitions of the concept. Definitions of self-advocacy make the concept prescriptive and suggest there are right and wrong ways to self-advocate (Hagan & Donovan, 2013b). The problem with this approach is the potential to essentialize women's expressions of control over their cancer experiences. As stated previously, characteristics of some cancers, including multiple recurrences and severe treatment aftereffects, may inhibit cancer survivors' abilities to actively self-advocate, per popular definitions of the term. For instance, ovarian cancer survivors whose disease has recurred prefer to defer treatment decisions to physicians because of increased trust in physicians, awareness of limited effective treatment options, and because they consider treatment a way to manage, rather than cure, the disease (Elit, et al., 2010). Thus, the blanket expectation that every cancer survivor should self-advocate in specific formats downplays differences in individual experiences and preferences.

Further, emphasis on self-advocacy shifts the responsibility for fighting cancer and staying strong and healthy onto the individual. Rigidly encouraging (and expecting) cancer survivors to assume responsibility for their health by making their voices and preferences for care known puts the burden of responsibility on survivors, suggesting that the community, including advocates and other cancer survivors, have made resources and support available and it is up to the individual survivor to access and utilize these. This supports notions of individualization of health, which feminist scholars continue to challenge. Individualization of health holds the individual/woman (not social and cultural systems) responsible for managing her own health (Dubriwny, 2013; Kissling, 2013; Fixmer-Oraiz, 2014). Deborah Lupton (1994) explores the concept by focusing on popular discourses that blame women for getting breast cancer for supposedly rejecting traditional feminine roles. Wilkinson and Kitzinger (1993) also problematize victim-blaming in alternative cancer self-care literature, arguing that this narrative about and attitude toward women's health is harmful as it places the blame on the individual for having cancer and thus expects the individual to take responsibility (through positive thinking) to overcome cancer.

Related to the personal responsibility consequence of self-advocacy is the notion of positive thinking, which also individualizes health and victimizes cancer survivors. There is increasing pressure on survivors to maintain a positive perspective about their health in order to effectively manage treatment symptoms and side effects. Positive thinking is emphasized because it is in line with societal values of self-control and increased self-esteem as a consequence of overcoming one's challenges (De Raeve, 1997). Hence, positive thinking and self-advocacy have become common concepts in the cancer self-help literature, are endorsed by society, promoted widely, and integrated into the vocabulary of cancer survivorship (Wilkinson & Kitzinger, 2000). Positive-thinking is pervasive in mainstream cancer discourses such that survivors apply the term to their experiences even when realities of their lives and health contradict its meanings; many cancer survivors hesitate to explicitly resist the think positive idiom even if they do not agree with it (Kitzinger, 2000; Wilkinson & Kitzinger, 2000). They use it vaguely as a "conversational idiom" to contribute to an ongoing conversation (Wilkinson & Kitzinger, 2000), similar to how idioms are used and responded to at face value (Kitzinger, 2000). Thinking positive can also be a strategy to talk about an emotionally laden topic such as cancer without burdening listeners; or a strategy to tone down negative emotional impacts of talking about cancer (Wilkinson & Kitzinger, 2000). Similarly, maintaining a positive attitude is a way for cancer survivors to articulate and make sense of their experiences and protect relational others, including spouses and children (McCreaddie, Payne & Froggatt, 2010). Thus, positive thinking in the cancer context has varied meanings for different people depending on context, individual circumstances, and stage of disease (McCreaddie, Payne & Froggatt, 2010).

However, scholars have criticized blanket use of the term and highlighted the implications for survivors. They suggest that over-emphasizing positive thinking promotes "false optimism" (De Raeve, 1997, p. 251) that communicates to cancer survivors that they can/should not entertain negative thoughts/emotions. Judy Z. Segal (2015) states she was offended, after her tenth radiation treatment for breast cancer, to see advice in the official magazine for the British Columbia Cancer Foundation, *Vim and Vigour,* about how cancer survivors can turn negative thoughts into positive ones. Segal is appalled because the advice does not reflect every person's cancer experience and also because encouraging cancer survivors to "improve your attitude" is insensitive and unhelpful (p. 218). Indeed, thinking positive is considered a "moral imperative" of cancer survivors; survivors are required to keep a positive outlook to get well (Wilkinson & Kitzinger, 2000; Wilkinson, 2001). The danger of this pervasive discourse is that outcomes of treatment are attributed to how well survivors are able to maintain a positive attitude following diagnosis and treatment (Wilkinson, 2001). This creates a perfect climate for individual responsibility, victim blaming and guilt. If thinking positive is seen as having the ability to ease disease progression (although having a positive attitude is not a sufficient condition for keeping cancer at bay; Hagan & Donovan, 2013a), it follows, then, that poor health outcome is the result of sufferers' failure to think positive (De Raeve, 1997). Emphasis on positive thinking can cause cancer survivors to feel guilty for not responding well to treatment as they believe their supposed negative attitude is responsible for their health outcomes (De Raeve, 1997). Indeed, some cancer survivors have internalized this understanding that they consider it their individual responsibility to maintain a positive attitude. They disguise their actual feelings and emotions in an effort not to be seen as weak and to not negate normative expectations of the cancer survivor as strong and heroic (Norberg et al., 2015). Survivors also consider it their responsibility to keep a positive attitude to protect relational others from negative responses to the cancer experience (De Raeve, 1997). As Samantha King (2006) points out, dominance of the "cure" and "optimism" narrative in breast cancer discourses suggests that positive attitude, strength of/by individual survivors, and large donations by corporate sponsors are the appropriate and effective means to fight the disease—a discourse that can alienate survivors who do not embrace the positive thinking concept (Sulik, 2011).

Recognizing the dangers of narrow emphasis on optimism, self-advocacy and positive thinking, this book suggests caution is exercised when promoting self-advocacy in the ovarian cancer context. This way, good intentions to encourage survivors to be actively involved in their health care do not inadvertently victimize them. Emphasizing positive thinking can be at the expense of openly acknowledging women's lived realities (Lorde, 1997). The lived reality of ovarian cancer is tough and the strength women demonstrate (regardless of the form and shape this takes) should be for individual survivors to determine.

It is also important to acknowledge that advocacy and self-advocacy may manifest concurrently in the case of ovarian cancer. It may be that in an effort to advocate for the disease that some survivors expressly embody self-advocacy (per popular definitions of the term); this may happen outside the medical setting when the disease is in remission. And, what may appear as non-self-advocacy may actually be how individual survivors choose to embody self-advocacy. Differences in experiences and expressions of advocacy and self-advocacy need to be encouraged and celebrated.

NOTES

1. Attributes of self-advocacy include possessing thoughts consistent with self-advocacy such as adjusting to cancer diagnosis and feeling empowered; taking actions for oneself, including navigating the healthcare system, making informed decisions, and practicing "mindful nonadherence"; and utilizing resources such as formal and informal support resources and using one's experience to support cancer awareness efforts (Hagan & Donovan, 2013b).
2. The OCC supports each survivor with $500 per year. This is an increase from the $250 it previously provided.
3. Avon has narrowed its focus on women's health issues to focus on breast cancer (King, 2006).
4. This is similar to influences of the women's health movement on the women's self-help movement. Taylor and Willigen (1996) suggest that organizing strategies of postpartum depression and breast cancer self-help groups, including provision of direct service, consciousness-raising, and lobbying, were direct influences of the women's health movement of the 1970s.
5. Other recipients of the grant were the American Red Cross and Autism Speaks.
6. The STS program was started in 2002 by Betty Reiser at the University of Medicine and Dentistry in New Jersey. The program was later adopted by the Ovarian Cancer Alliance. An evaluation of the STS program in Canada between 2006 and 2009 showed it has helped increased medical students' knowledge about survivors' perspectives on the disease (Fitch et al., 2011).

Chapter Seven

Afterword

Marrying the Personal and Medical to Improve Ovarian Cancer

I have examined the embodied experience of ovarian cancer from the perspectives of women who have lived with/through the disease, to have these women tell us what ovarian cancer survivorship is like. My investigation focused on different phases in the ovarian cancer trajectory, including diagnosis and treatment, secondary prevention and monitoring for recurrence, and management of recurrent disease (Committee on the State of the Science in Ovarian Cancer Research et al., 2016). I have also shed light on how social and cultural beliefs and norms about women's bodies and health impact how we come to understand ovarian cancer and survivors' communicative responses to the disease and treatments. By critically examining medical, social, and cultural discourses, norms, and standards that inhibit full appreciation of women's embodiments of ovarian cancer, I aimed to draw attention to a number of issues worth considering. Below, I suggest ways to move beyond system flaws to improve the disease experience, arguing primarily that the personal and medical/scientific need to be married to advance knowledge about ovarian cancer.

First, I argue that women's voices and lived experiences are indispensable in constructing knowledge about women's health. The number of women and families affected by ovarian cancer globally and the fact that the disease has been around for decades but scientific grasp on it is still limited, point to a need to re-assess how and where we are looking to for answers to the disease. Ovarian cancer is a disease specific to women; thus, women's personal experiences can significantly contribute to scientific efforts to understand the disease. It only makes sense not to exclude and/or by-pass women who embody the disease in attempts to understand it. In addition to the powerful evidence personal experience provides (Foss & Foss, 1994), survivors' personal accounts can help illuminate, contextualize, and give direction to scientific research about the disease. As I have discussed, many women and society at large lack in-depth knowledge about ovarian cancer. This is partly because of the dense, discipline-specific language used to report disease-related research; such language is inaccessible to lay people, including women to whom the disease pertains. Similarly, because of the biomedical discipline's emphasis on objectivity and scientific inquiry, methods of research and writing that prioritize subjective experiences are considered less rigorous and hence, are less appreciated. Because of their training many physicians and gynecologists by default value scientific research findings over personal experiences. I suggest this needs to change if we are committed to making headways in finding cure for the disease. Changing the trend and learning to listen to and value women's accounts of ovarian cancer will require deliberate and conscious effort on the part of physicians and society. It will require we consistently challenge and re-examine how we perceive women, their bodies, and health. Physicians and gynecologists need to learn to balance tenets of their trainings with the lived realities of survivors' experiences during each medical encounter. They need to consider their training as ongoing and constantly being improved through encounters with patients, meaning that women's subjective experiences are important to a better medical practice. This will require work, but it is attainable if physicians and gynecologists work with women as allies. Another key reason women's subjective voices are necessary is because statistics and mainstream information about ovarian cancer do not always corroborate women's lived experiences. And, women's lived experiences can challenge (and even enhance) the stories science constructs about women's bodies and health (Martin, 2001). To reiterate, listening to women's voices alone cannot magically solve all the issues and unknowns about the disease. But, as I suggested in chapter 2, listening to women's voices is significant to unlocking the puzzle about the disease and validating their experiences. This can be a step closer to challenging the status quo about science and medicine (as powerful and supposedly context- and value-free) and thereby, open up avenues to explore other possible meanings of the disease. Prioritizing one discourse (i.e., scientific/medical) over other equally important ones (i.e., personal experience) leads to minimization and neglect of the so-called less prominent discourses.

Second, survivors' voices are vital to the process as well as the outcomes. Focusing on the end result of scientific inquiry while ignoring injustices (to women) during the process can prove deleterious in the short- and long-term. Thus, I suggest that the scientific community recognizes women as allies in strides being made to understand the disease. Prioritizing scientific advancements over women's intimate experiences works to the disadvantage of women who alone suffer consequences for late diagnosis; and also to the advancement of knowledge about the disease. It disadvantages women by centralizing beliefs that science and medicine are the only means to getting a handle on ovarian cancer (the implication being that women need not bother to understand the disease) and that knowledge about the disease is attained top-down (from medical experts to women) and not the other way around. This rhetoric has somehow been effective in projecting ovarian cancer as beyond the grasp of lay people, and as I have explained, this undermines women's knowledge about their bodily experiences. Scientific ways of knowing (and claims about women's health) are neither absolute nor immune from cultural influences. Social and cultural contexts cannot be separated from efforts to understand ovarian cancer as these shape medical constructions of the disease and women's embodiments and interpretations of it. Yes, there is still a lot that is unknown about ovarian cancer even as scientific knowledge base about the disease keeps changing. For instance, we are learning that many ovarian cancers originate from the fallopian tubes, not the ovary, and that there are vast differences within and among the subtypes of the disease (Committee on the State of the Science in Ovarian Cancer Research et al., 2016). This means that each disease subtype will require different treatment regimen and will be embodied differently by women. Much as the scientific community is working hard to understand the disease and determine effective course of treatments (and we need to support their efforts and give them space to do their investigations), we also need to hold them accountable for their responsibility to women, to include them in the discovery process.

Third, representations of women's cancers (and other health issues) in popular culture and/or medical discourse need to be critically assessed. Language is powerful; it can shape how we think about an issue and highlight some aspects of an issue while concealing others. Similarly, discursive and visual representations of ovarian cancer can impact what society knows about the disease. Ovarian cancer has limited public visibility partly because the disease is construed as a medical mystery, because it usually has poor prognosis, and because of parts of the female body it is associated with (i.e., the ovaries and fallopian tubes). Popular rhetoric of lack of reliable screening for ovarian cancer and of who may be at risk also is implicative for public understanding of the disease. I suggest we become strategic in how we construct and represent the disease. This can take varied forms, including naming the disease when someone close to us or a public personality is affected by it. For instance, instead of saying "my aunt has cancer" we should say "my aunt has ovarian cancer." This will expose the public to the disease and add human faces to it. While US actress and director Angelina Jolie's public management of her BRCA mutation has brought attention to breast cancer and ovarian cancer (Troiano, Nantea & Cozzolino, 2017), she did not specifically name the type of cancer her mother had when explaining her family history of and predisposition to cancer in her 2013 op-ed in *The New York Times*. Jolie's mother died of ovarian cancer. In her 2015 op-ed, Jolie stated her mother had ovarian cancer only in her explanation as to why doctors recommended she removed her ovaries at age 39: "My mother's ovarian cancer was diagnosed when she was 49. I'm 39" (8). In my view, given the public and media influence Jolie commands, her failure to specifically name ovarian cancer in the 2013 op-ed is problematic. Because we do not often call ovarian cancer by its specific name, specifics of women cancers and their unique experiences are sometimes lost to the extent that people believe that if a woman has cancer, it must be breast cancer. For example, Martha Holmes (2006) narrates how due to limited public visibility of ovarian cancer, when she disclosed to her students that she had cancer "they look directly at my breasts, to see the absence; for most of them, women with cancer probably have breast cancer, and maybe a mastectomy" (p. 488). This suggests that we do more to put ovarian cancer on the public's radar, including calling it by its name.

Further, being strategic in how we construct and represent the disease requires that feminist, critical/cultural scholars, and others question and point out limitations in popular and medical representations of the disease. For instance, I noted in chapter two a need to challenge popular and scientific classifications of ovarian cancer risk factors as these blindside physicians and women supposedly not at risk. Along similar lines, it is imperative we continue to problematize limitations of ovarian cancer education efforts that ask women to know their bodies, eat healthy, and exercise to maintain an ideal body weight. While this approach seeks to give control over their health and bodies to women, it is limiting in that developing awareness about one's body is not the only break we need to advance knowledge about ovarian cancer. Even more problematic is how this approach promotes individual responsibility for health and obfuscates attention to larger issues and questions we should be addressing, such as inequality in access to quality health care. The concept of individual responsibility for health suggests that disease or risk of disease is an individual experience hence a responsibility of the individual to address such risk (Simpson, 2000). In reality, women can be (actually, they are) experts in their body knowledge; but until such knowledge is given the credence and attention it deserves, it is of minimal use and only frustrates women who want to take charge of their health care. Further, language of such education and awareness efforts focuses attention on women and their behavior (implying that women brought cancer on themselves by indulging in poor lifestyle choices and resisting societal control of their bodies by failing to have children early or give birth at all) and justifies drastic and dehumanizing treatment interventions (see Broom, 2001; Lupton, 1994). I suggest we broaden how we educate about the disease to include experiences that follow the standard symptom and disease pattern and those that do not. In this vein, I applaud efforts leaders of the Survivors Teaching Students (STS) program are making to improve medical and popular narratives about the disease. However, I find the format of the program problematic as it constricts diverse narratives about the disease.

The STS program provides ovarian cancer survivors with an opportunity to teach medical and nursing students about the disease using personal experience. The initiative is meant to strengthen opportunities for collaboration between survivors and the medical/scientific establishment—a collaboration that can prove invaluable given that ovarian cancer survivorship, including diagnosis and treatments, is a joint effort involving women, health care workers, and medical technologies. The STS program does not only help improve understanding about the disease from the perspectives of survivors; it can also provide avenues of closure for survivors as they explain the disease from their perspectives. It can be therapeutic for women to finally have a platform where their viewpoints are accepted and respected without question. However, it is important to realize that the STS program does not tell the entire story of ovarian cancer as it is not every survivor who is able (or willing) to participate. Women managing recurrent disease and those experiencing severe treatment aftereffects may choose to put their health first instead of participating in the STS program. For some, also, re-living traumatic events of diagnosis and treatments through the STS program can be stressful. Further, the STS program is structured such that women's narratives follow a strict format determined by the Ovarian Cancer Research Fund Alliance (OCRFA). The program is approximately an hour-long during which survivors share their stories by highlighting risks and symptoms of the disease and referral options for women suspected of having the disease. Women's stories follow a format provided by the OCRFA; stories are submitted for editing during a training session to meet time requirements (each woman has 7 minutes to tell her story) and for compliance with program guidelines (STS Handbook for Program Volunteers, 2017). Women cannot give opinions about a medical doctor or facility; they can only share information that is medically accurate to illustrate difficulty with early diagnosis of the disease (STS Handbook for Program Volunteers, 2017). The strict structure of the program can be disadvantageous in encouraging a standard narrative about the disease and restricting diverse presentations of survivors' stories, including stories that question the medical establishment (e.g., the STS program handbook states that volunteers who cannot comply with the program guidelines will not be allowed to participate). I would suggest to leaders of the program to consider ways to encourage survivors to tell their own stories without restrictions. Until women are supported to voice their experiences, including expressing anger and frustrations, the entire story of the disease will not be heard.

Related to broadening education and perspectives about the disease is a need to re-think meanings of terms such as "courage," "strength," and "control" as they pertain to ovarian cancer. Varied experiences of the disease reverse the meanings of these terms. As I have discussed, the nature of ovarian cancer means that women may look well and healthy when they are actually sick with cancer cells lurking in their bodies, and when they look weak and sick, that is when they are well. Jackie Stacey (1997) succinctly illustrates this point with photographs of herself before and after diagnosis and treatments for germ cell ovarian tumor (i.e., ovarian teratoma). She explains the first picture in which "the healthy, tanned body concealed a large and potentially lethal tumor" (p. 137) and the second where "The scarred and bloated body attracted sympathetic (and fearful, or just plain curious) gaze and yet it no longer housed a cancerous tumor" (p. 139). Similarly, Martha Holmes (2006) also compares photographs of herself before and after her ovarian cancer diagnosis. She says of the photograph before her diagnosis that even though "tumors were taking over my ovaries. . . . To most observers, although I am sick and in danger of becoming much sicker, I look more or less well" (p. 485). And about her second photograph taken six months after treatments when she was cancer-free she says, "I have no hair anywhere—no eyebrows, no eyelashes. I look faded, anxious, and simian, like a scrawny Yoda. . . . I may look weird, awful, and ill, but in this photo, I am well" (p. 485). These testimonies, together with examples presented in this book, point to a need to re-conceptualize popular notions of illness, health, strength, weakness, and beauty in the ovarian cancer context. I argue that women exhibit the uttermost strength during treatments when they appear weak and without some body parts (i.e., hair, ovary), and this needs to be highlighted in narratives about the disease. Instead of the healthy, young body being the standard against which the post-ovarian-cancer-treatment body is compared, we need to discard these supposed standards and appreciate each body in its own right and give credit to those bodies which have endured harsh medical treatments and are still living.

Along similar lines, there is a need to re-envision survivors' embodiments of treatments, including behaviors they exhibit that may come across as adherence to socially sanctioned identities and roles. Simply analyzing women's performances of "strong" and "healthy" as submission to hegemonic expectations of women and the ill indicates a failure to consider other implications of such identity performances, including the fluidity of identity negotiations. I argue that women perform these identities as active identity negotiation and uncertainty management strategies. They are looking out for themselves and relational others; their sense of inner security is tied to the well-being of relational others. The broader implications of connections between women's health and the health of their families need to be taken into consideration in interpreting women's communicative responses to treatments. I have explained that by performing socially-sanctioned identities as sick people during treatments, women exert control through compliance and by adopting "body-as-object" mindsets to endure treatments (Parton et al., 2017). This positions women as active agents in determining their own experiences by subverting mainstream meanings of words such as 'strength' and 'resilience' in embodiments of the disease.

Equally significant and deserving research attention are the experiences of non-heterosexual women (e.g., lesbian and bisexual women), disabled women, women from different cultural backgrounds, and others whose experiences of (ovarian) cancer are under-represented in the literature. The perspectives of these women are crucial in constructing a nuanced and holistic picture of the lived experience of cancer. There is limited research on cancer experiences of non-heterosexual women, for instance (Brown & Tracy, 2008). The few studies that focused on these women's experiences with cancer illustrate that the needs of these women (e.g., psychological and emotional and issues related to sexuality and social support) are not markedly different from those of their heterosexual colleagues. However, the manner in which these needs are experienced and satisfied (i.e., support to meet these needs) is different for non-heterosexual women than for their heterosexual counterparts (Hill & Holborn, 2015). For instance, in their study on sexual minority women's experiences of breast cancer and breast reconstruction, Rubin and Tanenbaum (2011) found that the majority of participants had breast reconstructions for similar reasons that heterosexual women subscribe to the procedure (e.g., to feel whole, look normal and to avoid external prostheses) and the explanations of those who chose not to get the procedure mirrored reasons women in general give for electing not to have breast reconstructions (e.g., to avoid additional surgery and pain). Rubin and Tanenbaum (2011) argue that sexual minority women's decisions to have breast reconstruction following cancer may be impacted more by influences of the "able-bodied gaze" than the male sexual gaze. Similarly, Arena and colleagues (2007) noted similarities in perceived available support and intrusive thoughts for lesbians and heterosexual women treated for breast cancer; but found that lesbians used adaptive coping strategies, including positive reframing, venting, and utilizing emotional support from friends, whereas heterosexual women engaged in denial. And, Boehmer, Miao and Ozonoff (2011) found that lesbian and bisexual women cancer survivors are more likely than heterosexual cancer survivors to report poor health. In another study, Boehmer and Case (2004) found that during medical encounters for breast cancer treatments, some sexual minority women did not disclose their sexual orientation for fear that they would be treated differently by physicians, among other reasons, and that both women who disclosed and those who did not disclose their sexual orientations were apprehensive during their encounters with physicians. No known study has focused exclusively on non-heterosexual women's experiences of ovarian cancer. Future research should address this gap in study.

Regarding women with physical disabilities, research suggests that many of them experience physical barriers in accessing care for cancer diagnosis and treatments. These barriers include difficulties using examination and diagnostic equipment and accessing hospital facilities (Iezzoni, Kilbridge & Park, 2010). Additionally, pre-existing disabilities (e.g., polio and multiple sclerosis) impact the quality of life of long-term cancer survivors (Becker, Kang & Stuifbergen, 2012). These physical challenges add another layer of stress to women's cancer experiences, necessitating a focused research agenda on these issues to better understand the perspectives of women with physical disabilities.

Also, culture undoubtedly has significant influences on the experience of illness and health. It determines people's perceptions about and understanding of cancer and management practices (Dein, 2004). For instance, in the African context cultural norms about feminine beauty, women, and their roles in society shape knowledge construction and management of issues related to women's health (Tetteh, 2017). Specifically in sub-Saharan Africa, because the breasts are associated with femininity and nurturance and because cultural standards of feminine beauty require women to be double-breasted, many women deny their risks of breast cancer due to potential physical effects of treatments (e.g., deformation from mastectomy). Thus, the disease is often diagnosed late (i.e., stages III or IV) and there is high disease-related mortality (Ajekigbe, 1991; Fregene & Newman, 2005; Ly et al., 2011). Ironically, these cultural standards and norms are inferred to construct a more positive image of (and thus high priority for) some women cancers than others. For instance, awareness and education efforts related to breast cancer are more prominent in some African countries than those for cervical cancer because of beliefs that cervical cancer is contracted through promiscuous sexual behavior (Reichenbach, 2002). These issues point to a need for communication and feminist scholars and others to continue investigating impacts of cultural beliefs and practices on women's cancer experiences.

Throughout this book, I have called for critical, reflective engagements with ovarian cancer and the medical, social, and cultural contexts in which the disease is experienced. Non-critical engagement with factors that directly and indirectly impact experiences of the disease limits our understanding of the disease and inhibits a thorough analysis of survivors' expressions of control and agency over their experiences. Uncritically engaging with these issues means privileging normative views about self-advocacy, a cancer survivor, and the female body, for example, over celebrating differences in women's individual experiences. It is significant that we recognize and accept differences in how each women chooses to embody ovarian cancer survivorship, including self-advocacy, treatment aftereffects, among others.

Supporting differences in women's embodiments of the disease could include changing conceptualizations of self-advocacy in the ovarian cancer context. As Gini and I discussed in chapter 6, we need to be careful when applying labels generated according to normative standards and ideals to women's experiences as these can discredit some experiences by classifying them as inadequate and can come across as collusion with hegemonic society to de-voice women's experiences.

Furthermore, professional ovarian cancer advocacy organizations should learn from failures of the breast cancer advocacy movement and scrutinize (or limit) financial support from large pharmaceutical and medical corporations. These organizations should constantly question whose interest this support serves: survivors or corporate entities? Monetary support the National Ovarian Cancer Coalition (NOCC) receives from corporate partners is alarming and can influence issues NOCC focuses on in its advocacy for survivors. Corporate sponsors can direct the agenda of cancer advocacy (see King, 2006).

Clearly, more needs to be done to support ovarian cancer survivors to fully embody the illness experience and to bring the disease to the public radar. This book is an attempt in that regard. I believe that we give society a fresh and balanced take on women's health issues when we take up issues considered prerogatives of the medical establishment, including ovarian cancer, and offer perspectives that center women's voices. To understand the disease and better appreciate and support the experiences of survivors, we need to move beyond the medical model to incorporate women's subjective perspectives, including conscious awareness of how ramifications of cultural constructions of the female body, normalized femininity, and beauty ideals manifest in the embodied experience of the disease. This can help improve knowledge about the disease (and women's health broadly) and give women and society the tools and information to engage in decisions and discussions about the disease.

Bibliography

Ajekigbe, A. T. (1991). Fear of mastectomy: The most common factor responsible for late presentation of carcinoma of the breast in Nigeria. *Clinical Oncology*, 3, 78–80.

Andersen, B. L. (2009). In sickness and in health: Maintaining intimacy after breast cancer recurrence. *The Cancer Journal, 15*(1), 70–73.

Andersen, M. R., Sweet, E., Lowe, K. A., Standish, L. J., Drescher, C. W., & Goff, B. A. (2012). Involvement in decision-making about treatment and ovarian cancer survivor quality of life. *Gynecologic Oncology, 124*(3), 465–470.

Anderson, M. S. & Johnson, J. (1994). Restoration of body image and self-esteem for women after cancer treatment: A rehabilitation strategy. *Cancer Practice, 2*(5), 345–349.

Anzaldúa, G. (1992). The new mestiza nation: A multicultural movement. In C. R. McCann & S. Kim (Eds.), *Feminist Theory Reader: Local and Global Perspectives* (277–284). New York: Routledge.

Atkins, L. (2016). Half the battle social support among women with cancer. *Qualitative Inquiry, 22*(4), 253–262.

Arena, P. L., Carver, C. S., Antoni, M. H., Weiss, S. Ironson, G. & Durán, R. E. (2007). Psychosocial responses to treatment for breast cancer among lesbian and heterosexual women. *Women & Health, 44*(2), 81–102. Doi: 10.1300/J013v44n02_05

Arnold, E. M. (1999). The cessation of cancer treatment as a crisis. *Social Work in Health Care, 29*, 21–38.

Babrow, S. A. (1992). Communication and problematic integration: Understanding diverging probability and value, ambiguity, ambivalence, and impossibility. *Communication Theory, 2*(2), 95–130.

Babrow, S. A. (2001). Uncertainty, value, communication, and problematic integration. *Journal of Communication, 51*(3), 553–573.

Babrow, A. S. & Matthias, M. S. (2009). Generally unseen challenges in uncertainty management: An application of problematic integration theory. In T. D. Afifi & W. A. Afifi (Eds.), *Uncertainty, information management, and disclosure decisions* (9–25). New York: Routledge.

Badr, H., & Taylor, C. L. C. (2006). Social constraints and spousal communication in lung cancer. *Psycho-Oncology, 15*, 673–683.

Bankhead, C. R., Collins, C., Stokes-Lampard, H., Rose, P., Wilson, S., Clements, A., Mant, D., Kehoe, S. T. & Austoker, J. (2008). Identifying symptoms of ovarian cancer: a qualitative and quantitative study. *British Journal of Obstetrics Gynecology, 115*, 1008–1014. Doi: 10.1111/j.1471–0528.2008.01772.x

Barker-Benfield, B. (1972). The spermatic economy: A nineteenth-century view of sexuality. *Feminist Studies 1* (1): 45–74.

Barry, M. J. & Edgman-Levitan, S. (2012). Shared decision making—The pinnacle of patient-centered care. *The New England Journal of Medicine, 366*(9), 780–781.

Bell, K. (2014). The breast-cancer-ization of cancer survivorship: Implications for experiences of the disease. *Social Science & Medicine 110*, 56–63.

Bell, L. (2014). Ethics and feminist research. In S. N. Hesse-Biber (Ed.) *Feminist Research Practice* (73–106). Thousand Oaks, CA: Sage.

Bell, K. & Ristovski-Slijepcevic, S. (2013). Cancer survivorship: Why labels matter. *Journal of Clinical Oncology, 31* (4), 409–411.

Bell, K. (2009). "If it almost kills you that means it's working": cultural models of chemotherapy expressed in a cancer support group. *Social Science & Medicine, 68* (1), 169–176.

Bodie, G. D. (2012). Task stressfulness moderates the effects of verbal person centeredness on cardiovascular activity: A dual-process account of the reactivity hypothesis. *Health Communication*, 27, 569–580.

Bodie, G. D. & Burleson, B. R. (2008). Explaining variations in the effects of supportive messages: A dual-process framework. *Annals of the International Communication Association*, 32(1), 355–398. Doi: 10.1080/23808985.2008.11679082

Bodie, G. D. & MacGeorge, E. L. (2015). Supportive communication theories: Dual process theory of supportive message outcomes and advice response theory. In D. O. Braithwaite & P. Schrodt (Eds.) *Engaging Theories in Interpersonal Communication: Multiple Perspectives* (129–141). Los Angeles, CA: Sage.

Boehmer, U. & Case, P. (2004). Physicians don't ask, sometimes patients tell: Disclosure of sexual orientation among women with breast carcinoma. *Cancer, 101*(8), 1882–1889.

Boehmer, U., Miao, X., & Ozonoff, A. (2011). Cancer survivorship and sexual orientation. *Cancer, 117*(16), 3796–3804.

Bordo, S. (1993). *Unbearable weight: Feminism, western culture, and the body*. Los Angeles, CA: University of California Press.

Bowes, D. E., Tamlyn, D. & Butler, L. J. (2002). Women living with ovarian cancer: Dealing with early death. *Health Care for Women International, 23*, 135–148.

Brashers, D. E., Haas, S. M. and Neidig, J. L. (1999). The patient self-advocacy scale: Measuring patient involvement in health care decision-making interactions. *Health Communication, 11*(2), 97–121.

Brashers, D. E. (2001). Communication and uncertainty management. *Journal of Communication, 51*(3), 477–497.

Brashers, D. E., Goldsmith, D. J., & Hsieh, E. (2002). Information seeking and avoiding in health contexts. *Human Communication Research, 28*, 258–271.

Brashers, D. E., Neidig, J. L. & Goldsmith, D. J. (2004). Social support and the management of uncertainty for people living with HIV or AIDS. *Health Communication, 16*(3), 305–331.

Brashers, D. E., Neidig, J. L., Haas, S. M., Dobbs, L. K., Cardillo, L. W. & Russell, J. A. (2000). Communication in the management of uncertainty: The case of persons living with HIV or AIDS. *Communication Monographs, 67*(1), 63–84.

Braun, V. & Clarke, V. (2006). Using thematic analysis in psychology. *Qualitative Research in Psychology, 3*, 77–101.

Bristow, R. E., Chang, J., Ziogas, A., Randall, L. M. & Anton-Culver, H. (2014). High-volume ovarian cancer care: Survival impact and disparities in access for advanced-stage disease. *Gynecologic Oncology, 132*. 403–410.

Broom, D. (2001) Reading breast cancer: reflections on a dangerous intersection. *Health* 5(2), 249–268.

Brown, J. P. & Tracy, J. K. (2008). Lesbians and cancer: An overlooked health disparity. *Cancer Causes and Control, 19*(10), 1009–1020.

Burleson, B. R. & Goldsmith, D. J. (1998). How the comforting process works: Alleviating emotional distress through conversationally induced reappraisals. In P. A. Andersen & L. K. Guerrero (Eds.), (245–280). *Handbook of Communication and Emotion: Research, Theory, and Contexts*. San Diego: CA: Academic Press

Callaghan, P. & Morrissey, J. (1993). Social support and health: A review. *Journal ofAdvanced Nursing, 18*, 203–210.

Carey, M. A. & Smith, M. W. (1994). Capturing the Group Effect in Focus Groups: A Special Concern in Analysis. *Qualitative Health Research, 4*(1), 123–127. Doi: 10.1177/104973239400400108.

Carter, R. R., DiFeo, A., Bogie, K., Zhang, G. & Sun, J. (2014). Crowdsourcing awareness: Exploration of the ovarian cancer knowledge gap through Amazon mechanical turk. *PLoS ONE, 9*(1): e85508. Doi:10.1371/journal.pone.0085508

Cass, I. & Karlan, B. Y. (2010). Ovarian cancer symptoms speak out—but what are they really saying? *Journal of the National Cancer Institute, 102*(4): 211–212. Doi: https://doi.org/10.1093/jnci/djp525

Cattapan, A., Hammond, K., Haw, J. & Tarasoff, L. A. (2014). Breaking the ice: Young feminist scholars of reproductive politics reflect on egg freezing. *International Journal of Feminist Approaches to Bioethics, 7*(2), 236–247. Doi: 10.1353/ijf.2014.0027

Caughlin, J. P., & Vangelisti, A. L. (2009). Why people conceal or reveal secrets: A multiple goals perspective. In T. Afifi & W. Afifi (Eds.), *Uncertainty, information management, and disclosure decisions: Theories and applications* (278–299). New York, NY: Routledge.

Caughlin, J. P., Mikucki-Enyart, S. L., Middleton, A. V., Stone, A. M. & Brown, L. E. (2011). Being open without talking about it: A rhetorical/normative approach to understanding topic avoidance in families after a lung cancer diagnosis. *Communication Monographs, 78*(4), 409–436.

Centers for Disease Control and Prevention (2010). Top 10 cancer sites: 2010, female, United States—All races. Retrieved from http://apps.nccd.cdc.gov/uscs/toptencancers.aspx#All

Cesario, K. S., Nelson, L. S., Broxson, A. & Cesario, A. L. (2010). Sword of Damocles cutting through the life stages of women with ovarian cancer. *Oncology Nursing Forum 37*(5), 609–617.

Charmaz, K. (1991). *Good days, bad days: The self in chronic illness and time*. New Brunswick, NJ: Rutgers University Press.

Charmaz, K. (1999). From the "sick role" to stories of self: Understanding the self in illness. In R. J. Contrada & R. D. Ashmore (Eds.), *Self, social identity, and physical health: Interdisciplinary explorations* (209–239). New York: Oxford University Press.

Clark, E. & Stovall, E. (1996). Advocacy: The cornerstone of cancer survivorship. *Cancer Practice 5*, 239–244.

Cleary, V. & Hegarty, J. (2011). Understanding sexuality in women with gynecological cancer. *European Journal of Oncology Nursing, 15*, 38–45.

Collins, P. H. (1986). Learning from the outsider within: The sociological significance of Black feminist thought. In A. M. Jaggar (2014, Ed.), *Just Methods: An interdisciplinary feminist reader* (308–320). Boulder, CO: Paradigm Publishers.

Collins, P. H. (1990). Defining Black Feminist thought. In C. R. McCann & S. Kim (Eds.), *Feminist Theory Reader: Local and Global Perspectives* (379–394). New York: Routledge.

Committee on the State of the Science in Ovarian Cancer Research, Board on Health Care Services, Institute of Medicine, National Academies of Sciences, Engineering, and Medicine (2016). *Ovarian Cancers: Evolving Paradigms in Research and Care* . Washington, DC: National Academy of Sciences.

Cooper, C. P., Polonec, L. & Gelb, C. A. (2010). Women's knowledge and awareness of gynecologic cancer: A multisite qualitative study in the United States. *Journal of Women's Health, 20*(4), 517–524.

Coward, D. D. & Kahn, D. L. (2005). Transcending breast cancer: Making meaning from diagnosis and treatment. *Journal of Holistic Nursing, 23(*3), 264–283. Doi: 10.1177/0898010105277649

Coyne, J. C. & Smith, D. A. F. (1991). Couples coping with a myocardial infarction: A contextual perspective on wives' distress. *Journal of Personality and Social Psychology, 61*(3), 404–412.

Dean, M. (2016). Celebrity health announcements and online health information seeking: An analysis of Angelina Jolie's preventative health decision. *Health Communication,* 31(6), 752–761. Doi: 10.1080/10410236.2014.995866

De Raeve L. (1997). Positive thinking and moral oppression in cancer care. *European Journal of Cancer Care, 6*, 249–256.

Dein, S. (2004). Explanatory models of and attitudes towards cancer in different cultures. *Lancet Oncology, 5*, 119–124.

Donovan-Kicken, E., Tollison, A. C. & Goins, E. S. (2012). The nature of communication work during cancer: Advancing the theory of illness trajectories. *Health Communication*, 27, 641–652. Doi: 10.1080/10410236.2011.629405.

Donovan-Kicken, E., Tollison, A. C. & Goins, E. S. (2011). A grounded theory of control over communication among individuals with cancer. *Journal of Applied Communication Research, 39*(3), 310–330. Doi: 10.1080/00909882.2011.585398.

Donovan-Kicken, E. & Caughlin, J. P. (2010). A multiple goals perspective on topic avoidance and relationship satisfaction in the context of breast cancer. *Communication Monographs, 77*, 231–256.

Dorgan, K. A., Duvall, K. L., Hutson, S. P., & Kinser, A. E. (2013). Mothered, mothering and motherizing in illness narratives: What women cancer survivors in southern central Appalachia reveal about mothering-disruption. *Journal of Appalachian Studies, 19*(1 & 2), 59–81.

Dorgan, K. A., Hutson, S. P., Duvall, K. L., Kinser, A. E. & Hall, J. M. (2014). Connecting place to disease and gender: Cohabitating morbidities in narratives of women cancer survivors in southern central Appalachia. *Women's Studies in Communication, 37*(3), 292–312. Doi: 10.1080/07491409.2014.950440

Doyal, L. (1983). Women, health and the sexual division of labor: A case study of the women's health movement in Britain. *International Journal of Health Services, 13*(3), 373–387.

Dubriwny, N. T. (2013). *The vulnerable empowered woman: Feminism, postfeminism, and women's health.* New Brunswick, NJ: Rutgers University Press.

Dubriwny, N. T. (2009). Constructing breast cancer in the news: Betty Ford and the evolution of the breast cancer patient. *Journal of Communication Inquiry,* 33(2), 104–125.

Duffey-Lind E. C., O'Holleran, E., Healey, M., Vettese, M., Diller, L. & Park, E. R. (2006). Transitioning to survivorship: A pilot study. *Journal of Pediatric Oncology Nursing, 23*(6), 335–343.

Ekman, I., Bergbom, I., Ekman, T., Berthold, H. & Mahsneh, S. M. (2004). Maintaining normality and support are central issues when receiving chemotherapy for ovarian cancer. *Cancer Nursing, 27*(3), 177–183.

Elit, L. Charles, C., Dimitry, S., Tedford-Gold, S., Gafni, A., Gold, I. & Whelan, T. (2010). It's a choice to move forward: Women's perceptions about treatment decision making in recurrent ovarian cancer. *Psycho-Oncology, 19*, 318–325.

Ellingson, L. L. (2004). Women cancer survivors: Making meaning of chronic illness, disability, and complementary medicine. In P. M. Buzzanell, H. Sterk & L. H. Turner (Eds.), *Gender in applied communication contexts* (79–98). Thousand Oaks, CA: Sage.

Ellis, C. (2007). Telling secrets, revealing lives: Relational ethics in research with intimate others. *Qualitative Inquiry, 13*, 3–29.

Faulkner, S. L. (2016). Cancer triptych. *Health Communication*, 1–4. Doi: 10.1080/10410236.2015.1020262.

Feichtinger, M. & Rodriguez-Wallberg, K. A. (2016). Fertility preservation in women with cervical, endometrial or ovarian cancers. *Gynecologic Oncology Research and Practice, 3*(8). Doi: 10.1186/s40661–016–0029–2

Ferrell, B., Smith, S. L., Cullinane, C. A. & Melancon, C. (2003). Psychological well-being and quality of life in ovarian cancer survivors. *Cancer,* 98(5), 1061–1071. Doi: 10.1002/cncr.11291

Ferrell, B., Smith, S. L., Cullinane, C. A. & Melancon, C. (2003). Symptom concerns of women with ovarian cancer. *Journal of Pain and Symptom Management, 25*(6), 528–538.

Ferrell, B. R., Smith, S. L., Juarez, G. & Melancon, C. (2003). Meaning of illness and spirituality in ovarian cancer survivors. *Oncology Nursing Forum, 30*(2), 249–257. Doi: 10.1188/03.onf.249–257

Fife, B. L. (1994). The conceptualization of meaning. *Social Science Medicine, 38*(2), 309–316.

Fitch, M. I., Gray, R. E. & Franssen, E. (2001). Perspectives on living with ovarian cancer: Older women's views. *Oncology Nursing Forum, 28*(9), 1433–1442.

Fitch, D., Deane, K., Howell, D. & Gray, R. E. (2002). Women's experiences with ovarian cancer: Reflections on being diagnosed. *Canadian Oncology Nursing Journal 12*(3), 152–168.

Fitch, M., McAndrew, A., Turner, F., Ross, E. & Pison, I. (2011). Survivors teaching students: Increasing awareness about ovarian cancer. *Canadian Oncology Nursing Journal/Revue canadienne de soins infirmiers en oncologie, 21*(1), 16–20.

Fixmer-Oraiz, Natalie. (2014). "(In)conceivable: Risky reproduction and the rhetorical labors of "Octomom." *Communication and Critical/Cultural Studies 11*(3): 231–249.

Floyd, K. & Ray, C. D. (2016). Thanks, but no thanks: Negotiating face threats when rejecting offers of unwanted social support. *Journal of Social and Personal Relationships*, 1–17. Doi: 10.1177/0265407516673161

Foss, K. A. & Foss, S. K. (1994). Personal experience as evidence in feminist scholarship. *Western Journal of Communication, 58*, 39–43.

Fredrickson, B. L. & Roberts, T-A. (1997). Objectification Theory: Toward understanding women's lived experiences and mental health risks. *Psychology of Women Quarterly, 21*(2),173–206.

Fregene, A., & Newman, L. A. (2005). Breast cancer in sub-Saharan Africa: How does it relate to breast cancer in African-American women? *Cancer 103*(8), 1540–1550.

Garofalo, J. P., Choppala, S., Hamann, H. A. & Gjerde, J. (2009). Uncertainty during the transition from cancer patient to survivor. *Cancer Nursing, 32*(4): E8–E14. Doi: 10.1097/ NCC.0b013e31819f1aab.

Gilbert, E., Ussher, J. M. & Perz, J. (2010). Renegotiating sexuality and intimacy in the context of cancer: The experiences of carers. *Archives of Sexual Behavior,* 39(4), 998–1009.

Gilbert, E., Ussher, J. M. & Perz, J. (2010a). Sexuality after breast cancer: A review. *Maturitas*, 66, 397–407.

Gilbert, E., Ussher, J. M., & Perz, J. (2011). Sexuality after gynecological cancer: A review of the material, intrapsychic, and discursive aspects of treatment on women's sexual wellbeing. *Maturitas*, 70, 42–57

Goldsmith, D. J. (2009). Uncertainty and communication in couples dealing with serious illness. In T. D. Afifi & W. A. Afifi (Eds.), *Uncertainty, information management, and disclosure decisions* (203–225). New York, NY: Routledge.

Goldsmith, D. J., Miller, L. E. & Caughlin, J. P. (2008). Openness and avoidance in couples communicating about cancer. *Annals of the International Communication Association, 31*(1), 62–115. Doi: 10.1080/23808985.2007.11679065

Greenberg, M. & Smith, R. A. (2016). Support seeking or familial obligation: An investigation of motives for disclosing genetic test results. *Health Communication, 31*(6), 668–678. Doi: 10.1080/10410236.2014.989384

Gubar, S. (2012). *Memoir of a debulked woman*. New York, NY: W.W. Norton & Company.

Hagan, T. L., & H. S. Donovan (2013a). Ovarian cancer survivors' experiences of self-advocacy: A focus group study. *Oncology Nursing Forum*, 40(2), 140–147.

Hagan, T. L. & H. S. Donovan (2013b). Self-advocacy and cancer: A concept analysis. *Journal of Advanced Nursing*, 69(10), 2348–2359.

Hagan, T. L. & Medberry, E. (2016). Patient education vs. patient experiences of self-advocacy: Changing the discourse to support cancer survivors. *Journal of Cancer Education, 31*, 375–381. Doi: 10.1007/s13187–015–0828-x

Happe, K. E. (2006). Heredity, gender and the discourse of ovarian cancer. *New Genetics and Society, 25*(2), 171–196. Doi: 10.1080/14636770600855226

Happe, E. K. (2013). Genetic testing, cancer risk, and Angelina Jolie's choice. *From the Square*. http://www.fromthesquare.org/genetic-testing-cancer-risk-and-angelina-jolies-choice/#.V9mFDZMrJBx

Happe, K. E. (2017). Genetics and Epigenetics. In S. Alaimo (Ed.) *Gender: Matter* (347–359). Farmington Hills, MI: Macmillan.

Hallowell, N. (2006). Varieties of suffering: Living with the risk of ovarian cancer. *Health, Risk & Society,* 8(1), 9–26.

Hallowell, N., Arden-Jones, A., Eeles, R., Foster, C., Lucassen, A., Moynihan, C. & Watson, M (2006). Guilt, blame and responsibility: men's understanding of their role in the transmission of BRCA1/2 mutations within their family. *Sociology of Health & Illness* 28(7), 969–988. Doi: 10.1111/j.1467–9566.2006.00515.x

Hallowell, N. & Lawton, J. (2002). Negotiating present and future selves: Managing the risk of hereditary ovarian cancer by prophylactic surgery. *Health: An Interdisciplinary Journal for the Social Study of Health, Illness and Medicine, 6*(4), 423–443.

Hawkins, Y., Ussher, J., Gilbert, E., Perz, J., Sandoval, M. & Sundquist, K. (2009). Changes in sexuality and intimacy after the diagnosis and treatment of cancer: The experience of partners in a sexual relationship with a person with cancer. *Cancer Nursing, 32*(4), 271–280.

Hawkins, N. A., Cooper, C. P., Saraiya, M., Gelb, C. A. & Polonec, L. (2011). Why the Pap test? Awareness and use of the Pap test among women in the United States. *Journal of Women's Health, 20*(4), 511–515.

Hayden, S. (2009). Revitalizing the debate between life and choice: The 2004 march for women's lives. *Communication and Critical/Cultural Studies,* 6(2), 111–131.

Hecht, M. L. (1993) 2002—a research odyssey: Toward the development of a communication theory of identity. *Communication Monographs, 60*(1), 76–82. Doi: 10.1080/03637759309376297

Hesse-Biber, S. (2014). A re-invitation to feminist research. In S. N. Hesse-Biber (Ed.) *Feminist Research Practice* (1–13). Thousand Oaks, CA: Sage.

Hewitt, M., Greenfield, S. & Stovall, E. (2006). *From cancer patient to cancer survivor: Lost in transition.* Washington, DC: The National Academies Press.

Hill, A. (2016). Breast cancer's rhetoricity: bodily border crisis and bridge to corporeal solidarity. *Review of Communication,* 16(4), 281–298. Doi: 10.1080/15358593.2016.1207347.

Hill, G. & Holborn, C. (2015). Sexual minority experiences of cancer care: A systematic review. *Journal of Cancer Policy, 6,* 11–22.

Hipkins, J., Whitworth, M., Tarrier, N. & Jayson, G. (2004). Social support, anxiety and depression after chemotherapy for ovarian cancer: A prospective study. *British Journal of Health Psychology, 9,* 569–581.

Holmes, S. M. (2006). "Pink ribbons and public private parts: On not imagining ovarian cancer." *Literature and Medicine, 25,*(2), 475–501. Doi: 10.1353/lm.2007.0005

Holmes, S. M. (2011). After Sontag: Reclaiming metaphor. *Genre,* 44(3), 263–276. Doi: 10.1215/00166928–1407594

Howell, D., Fitch, M. I. & Deane, K. A. (2003). Impact of ovarian cancer perceived by women. *Cancer Nursing, 26*(1), 1–9.

Hoffman, B. and Stovall, E. (2006). Survivorship perspectives and advocacy. *Journal of Clinical Oncology, 24*(32), 5154–5159. Doi: 10.1200/JCO.2006.06.5300.

Howlader, Nadia, A. M. Noone, M. Krapcho, J. Garshell, D. Miller, S. F. Altekruse, C. L. Kosary et al. (2015). *SEER cancer statistics review, 1975–2012.* Bethesda, MD: National Cancer Institute.

Hunt, A. (May, 2007). Quest Diagnostics celebrates 50th anniversary, grants NOCC with $50K. National Ovarian Cancer Coalition. Retrieved May 17, 2017 from http://ovarian.org/about-ovarian-cancer/what-are-the-signs-a-symptoms/417-quest-diagnostics-celebrates-50th-anniversary-grants-nocc-with-50k.

Iezzoni, L. I., Kilbridge, K. & Park, E. R. (2010). Physical access barriers to care for diagnosis and treatment of breast cancer among women with mobility impairments. *Oncology Nursing Forum, 37*(6), 711–717. Doi: 10.1188/10.ONF.711–717

Institute of Medicine (2013). *Delivering high-quality cancer care: Charting a new course for a system in crisis.* Washington, DC: The National Academies Press.

Jacobs, I. Davis, A. P., Bridges, J., Stabile, I., Fay, T., Lower, A., Grudzinskas, J. G., & Oram, D. (1993). Prevalence screening for ovarian cancer in postmenopausal women by CA 125 measurement and ultrasonography. *British Medical Journal, 306*(6884), 1030–1034.

Jaggar, A. M. (2013). Introduction: The project of feminist methodology. In A. M. Jaggar (2014, Ed.), *Just Methods: An interdisciplinary feminist reader* (vii–xiii). Boulder, CO: Paradigm Publishers.

Jolie, Angelina. (2013). My Medical Choice. *The New York Times.* http://www.nytimes.com/2013/05/14/opinion/my-medical-choice.html?_r=4&\&#h[IwtIct,1

Jolie. Angelina. (2015). Angelina Jolie Pitt: Diary of a Surgery. *The New York Times.* http://www.nytimes.com/2015/03/24/opinion/angelina-jolie-pitt-diary-of-a-surgery.html?_r=0

Jones, S. M. (2004). Putting the person into person-centered and immediate emotional support: Emotional change and perceived helper competence as outcomes of comforting in helping situations. *Communication Research, 32*, 338–360. Doi: 10.1177/0093650204263436

Jung, E. & Hecht, M. L. (2004). Elaborating the communication theory of identity: Identity gaps and communication outcomes. *Communication Quarterly, 52*(3), 265–283. Doi: 10.1080/01463370409370197

Kaplan, S. (2015). Angelina Jolie reveals preventive surgery to remove ovaries, fallopian tubes. *The Washington Post.* Reviewed from https://www.washingtonpost.com/news/morning-mix/wp/2015/03/24/angelina-jolie-undergoes-preventative-surgery-to-remove-her-ovaries/?utm_term=.8a84d58e897d

Kasper, A. S. (1995). The social construction of breast loss and reconstruction. *Women's Health: Research on Gender, Behavior, and Policy, 1*(3), 197–219.

Kayser, K., Watson, L. E. & Andrade, J. T. (2007). Cancer as a "we-disease": Examining the process of coping from a relational perspective. *Families, Systems, & Health, 25*(4), 404–418.

Kernan, W. D. & Lepore, S. J. (2009). Searching for and making meaning after breast cancer: Prevalence, patterns, and negative affect. *Social Science Medicine 68*, 1176–1182.

King, S. (2006). *Pink Ribbons, Inc.: Breast Cancer and the Politics of Philanthropy* Minneapolis, MN: University of Minnesota Press.

Kitzinger, C. (2000). How to resist an idiom. *Research on Language and Social Interaction, 33*(2), 121–154

Kitzinger, J. (1995). Introducing focus groups. *British Medical Journal, 311*, 299–302.

Kissling, E. A. (2013). Pills, Periods, and Postfeminism: The new politics of marketing birth control. *Feminist Media Studies,* 13(3), 490–504.

Kluger, J., & Park, A. (2013). The Angelina Jolie effect. *Time.* http://www.lang.osakau.ac.jp/~tabata/ENG2012/2013b_The_Angelina_Effect.pdf

Knobf, M. T. (2007). Psychosocial responses in breast cancer survivors. *Seminars in Oncology Nursing*, 23(1), 71–83.

Koczwara, B. & Ward, P. (2014). Response to Bell, K., The breast-cancer-ization of cancer survivorship: Implications for experiences of the disease. *Social Science & Medicine, 128*, 324–343.

Krychman, M. & Millheiser, L. S. (2013). Sexual Health Issues in Women with Cancer. *The Journal of Sexual Medicine*, 10(S1), 5–15.

Lalwani, A., Shanbhogue, A. K. P., Vikram, R., Nagar, A., Jagirdar, J. & Prasad, S. R. (2010). Current update on borderline ovarian neoplasms. *American Journal of Roentgenology, 194*, 330–336. Doi:10.2214/AJR.09.3936

Langellier, M. K., and C. F. Sullivan. (2003). "Breast talk in breast cancer narratives." *Qualitative Health Research* 8 (1): 76–94.

Lee, V., Cohen, S. R., Edgar, L., Laizner, A. M. & Gagnon, A. J. (2004). Clarifying "meaning" in the context of cancer research: A systematic literature review. *Palliative and Supportive Care, 2,* 291–303.

Lethborg, C. E., Kissane, D., Burns, W. I. & Snyder, R. (2000). "Cast adrift": The experience of completing treatment among women with early stage breast cancer. *Journal of Psychosocial Oncology, 18*(4), 73–90.

Leopold, E. (1999). *A darker ribbon: Breast cancer, women, and their doctors in the twentieth century.* Beacon Press: Boston: MA.

Levinson, W., Kao, A., Kuby, A. & Thisted, R. A. (2005). Not all patients want to participate in decision making: A national study of public preferences. *Journal of General Internal Medicine, 20*(6), 531–535.

Lippman, A. (1999). Choice as a risk to women's health. *Health, Risk & Society,* 1(3), 281–291.

Lippman, A. (1991). Prenatal genetic testing and screening: Constructing needs and reinforcing inequalities. *American. Journal of Law & Medicine,* 17, 15–50.

Little, M., Paul, K., Jordens, C. F., & Sayers, E. J. (2002). Survivorship and discourses of identity. *Psycho-Oncology, 11*(2), 170–178.

Lockwood, G. (2002). Politics, ethics and economics: Oocyte cryopreservation in the UK. *Reproductive BioMedicine Online, 6*(2), 151–153.

Lockwood-Rayermann, S. (2006). Survivorship issues in ovarian cancer: A review. *Oncology Nursing Forum, 33*(3), 553–562.

Lupton, D. (1994). Femininity, responsibility and the technological imperative: Discourse on breast cancer in the Australian press. *International Journal of Health Services,* 24(1), 73–89.

Ly, M., Antoine, M., Andre, F., Callard, P., Bernaudin, J. F., & Diallo D. A. (2011). Breast cancer in sub-Saharan African women: Review. *Bulletin du Cancer, 98*(7), 797–806. Retrieved from http://dx.doi.org/10.1684/bdc.2011.1392

Macilwain, C. (2015). Change the cancer conversation. *Nature,* 520(7545), 7–7.

Marieskind, H. (1975). The women's health movement. *International Journal of Health Services, 5*(2), 217–223.

Markman, M. & Malviya, V. (2008). An example of ovarian cancer as a "chronic disease process"—11-year survival with multiple treatments for recurrent and progressive disease. *Case reports in Oncology, 1*(1), 1–4.

Martin, E. (1991). The egg and the sperm: How science has constructed a romance based on stereotypical male-female roles. *Signs,* 16(3), 485–501.

Martin, E. (2001). *The women in the body: A cultural analysis of reproduction.* Boston, MA: Beacon Press.

Martin, L. T., Schonlau, M., Haas, A., Derose, K. P., Rosenfeld, L., Buka, S. L. & Rudd, R. (2011). Patient activation and advocacy: Which literacy skills matter most? *Journal of Health Communication,* 16(Sup3), 177–190. Doi: 10.1080/10810730.2011.604705

Martin, S. C. (2016). The experience and communicative management of identity threats among people with Parkinson's disease: Implications for health communication theory and practice. *Communication Monographs, 83*(3), 303–325. Doi: 10.1080/03637751.2016.1146407

McCallum, M., Lefebvre, M., Jolicoeur, L., Maheu, C., & Lebel, S. (2012). Sexual health and gynecological cancer: Conceptualizing patient needs and overcoming barriers to seeking and accessing services. *Journal of Psychosomatic Obstetrics & Gynecology,* 33(3), 135–142. Doi: 10.3109/0167482X.2012.709291

McCreaddie, M., Payne, S. & Froggatt, K. (2010). Ensnared by positivity: A constructivist perspective on "being positive" in cancer care. *European Journal of Oncology Nursing, 14,* 283–290.

McKenzie, H. & Crouch, M. (2004). Discordant feelings in the life-world of cancer survivors. *Health: An Interdisciplinary Journal for the Social Study of Health, Illness and Medicine, 8*(2), 139–157.

McKinley, E. D. (2000). On being a patient: Under toad days: Surviving the uncertainty of cancer recurrence. *Annals of Internal Medicine, 133*(6), 479–480.

Mead, E. L., Doorenbos, A. Z., Javid, S. H., Haozous, E. A., Alvord, L. A., Flum, D. R., & Morris, A., M. (2013). Shared decision-making for cancer care among racial and ethnic minorities: A systematic review. *American Journal of Public Health, 103*(12), e15–e29.

Michel, A. (2014). Beautiful Disease: The story of Angelina Jolie's mastectomy in the American media. *Marquette University.* Retrieved from http://epublications.marquette.edu/cgi/viewcontent.cgi?article=1013&context=dittman

Miller, L. E. (2015). "People don't understand that it is not easy being a cancer survivor": Communicating and negotiating identity throughout cancer survivorship. *Southern Communication Journal, 80*(1), 1–19.

Miller, L. E. & Coughlin, J. P. (2013). "We're going to be survivors": Couples' identity challenges during and after cancer treatment. *Communication Monographs, 80*(1), 63–82.

Miller, L. E. (2014b). Communication dilemmas in the context of cancer: Survivors' and partners' strategies for communicating throughout survivorship. *Issues in Mental Health Nursing, 35*(12), 914–923.

Miller, L. E., & Caughlin, J. P. (2013). "We're going to be survivors": Couples' identity challenges during and after cancer treatment. *Communication Monographs, 80*(1), 63–82.

Mishel, M. H. & Braden, C. J. (1987). Uncertainty: A mediator between support and adjustment. *Western Journal of Nursing Research, 9*(1), 43–57.

Morgan, D. L. (1996). Focus Groups. *Annual Review of Sociology, 22,* 129–152.

National Ovarian Cancer Coalition (n.d.). *Mission and Vision of NOCC.* Retrieved from http://ovarian.org/about-us/missionvision

National Cancer Institute, National Institutes of Health & U.S. Department of Health and Human Services (2012). Gynecologic cancers portfolio. Retrieved from https://www.icrpartnership.org/Publications/ICRP_GYN_analysis.pdf

National Ovarian Cancer Coalition (n.d.). Mission & Vision of NOCC. Retrieved from http://ovarian.org/about-us/missionvision

Norberg, M., Magnusson, E., Thyme, K. E., Åström, S., Lindh, J. & Öster, I. (2015). Breast cancer survivorship—Intersecting gendered discourses in a 5-year follow-up study. *Health Care for Women International*, 36, 617–633. Doi: 10.1080/07399332.2015.1017640

O'Hair, D., Villagran, M. M., Wittenberg, E., Brown, K., Ferguson, M. Hall, H. T. and Doty, T. (2003). Cancer survivorship and agency model: Implications for patient choice, decision making, and influence. *Health Communication, 15*(2), 193–202.

Ozga, M., Aghajanian, C., Myers-Virtue, S., McDonnell, G., Jhanwar, S., Hichenberg, S. & Sulimanoff, I. (2015). A systematic review if ovarian cancer and fear of recurrence. *Palliative and Supportive Care, 13*, 1771–1780. Doi: 10.1017/S1478951515000127

Park, C. L. (2010). Making sense of the meaning literature: An integrative review of meaning making and its effects on adjustment to stressful life events. *Psychological Bulletin, 136*(2), 257–301.

Parton, C. M., Ussher, J. M. & Perz, P. (2015). Women's construction of embodiment and the abject sexual body after cancer. *Qualitative Health Research*, 1–14. Doi: 10.1177/1049732315570130

Parton, C., Ussher, J. M. & Perz, J. (2017). The medical body: Women's experiences of sexual embodiment across the cancer illness trajectory. *Women's Reproductive Health, 4*(4), 46–60.

Peek, M. E., Gorawara-Bhat, R., Quinn, M. T., Odoms-Young, A., Wilson, S. C. & Chin, M. H. (2013). Patient trust in physicians and shared decision-making among African-Americans with diabetes. *Health Communication, 28*, 616–623. Doi: 10.1080/10410236.2012.710873

Petersen, L., Kruckek, A., & Shaffner, A. (2003). Gender roles and the family life cycle: The case of women with cancer. *Journal of Feminist Family Therapy*, 15, 99–119. Doi: 10.1300/J086v15n02_07

Petronio, S. & Durham, W. T. (2015). Communication Privacy Management Theory: Significance for interpersonal communication. In L. A. Baxter and D. O. Braithwaite (Eds.), *Engaging Theories in Interpersonal Communication: Multiple Perspectives* (2nd, 335–347). Thousand Oaks, CA: Sage.

Prat, J. (2014). Staging classification for cancer of the ovary, fallopian tube, and peritoneum. *International Journal of Gynecology and Obstetrics, 124*(1), å1–5

Price, B. (1998). Cancer: Altered body image. *Nursing Standard, 12*(21), 49–55.

Rainbow, P. "Artificiality and enlightenment: From sociobiology to biosociality." In J. Crary and S. Kwinter (Eds.), *Incorporations* (234–252). New York, NY: Zone.

Reb, M. A. (2007). Transforming the death sentence: Elements of hope in women with advanced ovarian cancer. *Oncology Nursing Forum,* 34(6), E70–E81.

Reichenbach, L. (2002). The politics of priority setting for reproductive health: Breast and cervical cancer in Ghana. *Reproductive Health Matters, 10*(20), 47–58.

Rossing, M. A., Wicklund, K. G., Cushing-Haugen, K. L. & Weiss, N. S. (2010). Predictive value of symptoms for early detection of ovarian cancer. *Journal of the National Cancer Institute, 102*(4), 222–229. Doi: 10.1093/jnci/djp500

Rubin, L. R. & Tanenbaum, M. (2011). "Does that make me a woman?": Breast cancer, mastectomy, and breast reconstruction decisions among sexual minority women. *Psychology of Women Quarterly, 35*(3), 401–414. Doi: 10.1177/0361684310395606

Ruzek, S. B. & Becker, J. (1999). The women's health movement in the United States: From grassroots activism to professional agendas. *Journal of the American Medical Women's Association,* 54(1), 4–8.

Salander, P. (2001). Bad news from the patient's perspective: An analysis of the written narratives of newly diagnosed cancer patients. *Social Science & Medicine, 55,* 721–732.

Sekse, R. J. T., Gjengedal, E. & Råhem, M. (2013). Living in a changed female body after gynecological cancer. *Health Care for Women International*, 34,14–33. Doi: 10.1080/07399332.2011.645965

Schaefer, C., Coyne, J. C. & Lazarus, R. S. (1981). The health-related functions of socialsupport. *Journal of Behavioral Medicine, 4*(4), 381–406.

Schink, J. C. (1999). Current initial therapy of stage III and IV ovarian cancer: Challenges for managed care. *Seminars in Oncology, 26*(1), 2–7.

Schultz, W. C. M. & van de Wiel, H. B. M. (2003). Sexuality, intimacy, and gynecologic cancer. *Journal of Sex and Marital Therapy, 29*(S), 121–128.

Semmer, N. K., Elfering, A., Jaobshagen, N., Perrot, T. Beehr, T. A., & Boos, N. (2008). The emotional meaning of instrumental social support. *International Journal of Stress Management, 15*(3), 235–251. Doi: 0.1037/1072–5245.15.3.235.

Shih, I. & Kurman, R. J. (2004). Ovarian tumorigenesis: A proposed model based on morphological and molecular genetic analysis. *American Journal of Pathology, 164*(5), 1511–1518.

Silva, T. V. (2011). Lost choices and eugenic dreams: Wrongful birth lawsuits in popular news narratives. *Communication and Critical/Cultural Studies,* 8(1), 22–40.

Simmons, A. R., Baggerly, K. & Bast, R. C. (2013). The emerging role of HE4 in the evaluation of advanced epithelial ovarian and endometrial carcinomas. *Oncology (Williston Park), 27*(6), 548–556.

Skaggs, B. G. & Barron, C. R. (2006). Searching for meaning in negative events: Concept analysis. *Journal of Advanced Nursing, 53*(5), 559–570.

Smith D. (1974). Women's perspective as a radical critique of sociology. In A. M. Jaggar (2014, Ed.), *Just Methods: An interdisciplinary feminist reader* (39–43). Boulder, CO: Paradigm Publishers.

Stacey, J. (1997). *Teratologies: A cultural Study of cancer*. New York, NY: Routledge.

Staller, K. M. & Buch, E. D. (2014). What is feminist ethnography? In S. N. Hesse-Biber (Ed.) *Feminist Research Practice* (107–144). Thousand Oaks, CA: Sage.

Stead, M. L., Fallowfield, L., Brown, J. M. & Selby, P. (2001). Communication about sexual problems and sexual concerns in ovarian cancer: Qualitative study. *British Medical Journal, 323,* 836–837.

Stewart, D. E., Wong, F., Duff, A., Melancon, C. H. & Cheung, A. M. (2001). "What doesn't kill you makes you stronger": An ovarian cancer Survivor Survey. *Gynecologic Oncology*, 83, 537–542. Doi: 10.1006/gyno.2001.6437.

Sulik, G. A. (2007a). On the receiving end: Women, caring, and breast cancer. *Qualitative Sociology, 30*(3), 297–314.

Sulik, G. A. (2007b). The balancing act: Care work for the self and coping with breast cancer. *Gender and Society, 12*(6), 857–877.

Sulik, A. G. (2011). *Pink ribbon blues: How breast cancer culture undermines women's health.* New York, NY: Oxford University Press.

Sunnybrook Health Sciences Center. 2014. "'*Angelina Effect*' *on breast cancer genetic screening*." http://sunnybrook.ca/media/item.asp?c=1&i=1174&page=33939&f=angelina-jolie-breast-cancer-genetic-screening

Sun, C. C., Ramirez, P. T. & Bodurka, D. C. (2007). Quality of life for patients with epithelial ovarian cancer. *Clinical Oncology, 4*(1), 18–29.

Survivors Teaching Students: Saving Women's Lives® (2017). Handbook for Program Volunteers. *Ovarian Cancer Research Fund Alliance.*

Taylor, V. & Willigen M. V. (1996). Women's self-help and the reconstruction of gender: The postpartum support and breast cancer movements. *Mobilization: An International Journal, 1*(2), 123–142.

Temple, S. V. (2002). The advocacy movement in gynecologic oncology. *Seminars in Oncology Nursing, 18*(3), 231–235.

Tetteh, D. A. (2017). The breast cancer fanfare: Sociocultural factors and women's health in Ghana. *Health Care for Women International, 38*(4), 316–333

Thompson, S. C. & Pitts, J. (1993). Factors relating to a person's ability for find meaning after a diagnosis with cancer. *Journal of Psychosocial Oncology, 11*(3), 1–21. Doi: 10.1300/J077V11N03_01.

Trivers, K. F., Patterson, J. R., Roland, K. B. & Rodriguez, J. L. (2013). Issues of ovarian cancer survivors in the USA: A literature review. *Support Care Cancer, 21*, 2889–2898. Doi: 10.1007/s00520–013–1893–5

Troianoa, G., Nantea, N. & Cozzolino, M. (2017). The Angelina Jolie effect – Impact on breast and ovarian cancer prevention: A systematic review of effects after the public announcement in May 2013. *Health Education Journal,* 76(6), 707 –715.

Twombly, R. (2007). Cancer killer may be "silent" no more. *Journal of the National Cancer Institute, 99*(18), 1359–1361.

Uchino, B. V. (2004). *Social support and physical health: Understanding the health consequences of relationships*. Nashville, TN: Yale University Press.

Umberson, D. & Montez, J. K. (2010). Social Relationships and Health: A Flashpoint for Health Policy. *Journal of Health and Social Behavior, 51*(S), S54-S66. Doi: 10.1177/0022146510383501

Umberson, D., Crosnoe, R. & Reczek, C. (2010). Social Relationships and Health Behaviors across the Life Course. *Annual Review of Sociology, 36*, 139–157. Doi: 10.1146/annurev-soc-070308–120011

Ussher, M. J. (1989). *The psychology of the female body*. New York, NY: Routledge.

Ussher, J. M. (2006). *Managing the Monstrous Feminine: Regulating the Reproductive Body.* London: Routledge.

Vaz, A. F., Pinto-Neto, A. M., Conde, D. M., Costa-Paiva, L., Morais, S. S., & Esteves, S. B. (2007). Quality of life of women with gynecologic cancer: Associated factors. *Archives of Gynecology and Obstetrics, 276*(6), 583–589.

Ward, S. E., Heidrich, S. M. & Donovan, H. S. (2007). An update on the representational approach to patient education. *Journal of Nursing Scholarship, 39*(3), 259–265. Doi: 10.1111/j.1547–5069.2007.00178.x.

Wilkinson, S. (2001). Breast cancer: Feminism, representations and resistance—a commentary on Dorothy Broom's "Reading breast cancer." *Health, 5*(2): 269–277

Wilkinson, S. & Kitzinger, C. (2000). Thinking differently about positive thinking: A discursive approach to cancer patients' talk. *Social Science and Medicine, 50*, 797–811.

Wilkinson, S. & Kitzinger, C. (1993). Whose breast is it anyway? A feminist consideration of advice and "treatment" for breast cancer. *Women's Studies International Forum, 16*(3), 229–238.

Wilmoth, M. C. & Spinelli, A. (2000). Sexual implications of gynecologic cancer treatments. *Journal of Obstetric, Gynecologic, and Neonatal Nursing, 29*(4), 413–421.

Woods, N. F. (1987). Toward a holistic perspective of human sexuality: Alterations in health and nursing diagnoses. *Holistic Nursing Practice, 1*(4), 1–11.

Wright, K. B., Frey, L. & Sopory, P. (2007). Willingness to communicate about health as an underlying trait of patient self-advocacy: The development of the willingness to communicate about health (WTCH) measure. *Communication Studies, 58*(1), 35–51.

Yee, S., Abrol, K., McDonald, M., Tonelli, M. & Liu, K. E. (2012). Addressing oncofertility needs: Views of female cancer patients in fertility preservation. *Journal of Psychosocial Oncology, 30*(3), 331–346.

Zebrack, B. J. (2000). Cancer survivor identity and quality of life. *Cancer practice*, *8*(5), 238–242.

Zhang, A. Y. & Siminoff, L. A. (2003). Silence and cancer: Why do families and patients fail to communicate? *Health Communication, 15*(4), 415–429.

Zoller, H. M. (2005). Health activism: Communication theory and action for social change. *Communication Theory, 15*(4), 341–364.

Zoller, H. M. (2004). NIH develops consensus statement on ovarian cancer. *American Family Physician, 50(1), (Special Medical Reports), 213–216.*

Zoller, H. M. (n.d.). "The Angelina Jolie effect: Survey finds celebrity health choices may impact important consumer health decisions." Accessed June 3, 2013. http://bc5project.com/survey.pdf

Index

About the Author

Dinah A. Tetteh, PhD, is an assistant professor in the Department of Communication at Arkansas State University.

www.ingramcontent.com/pod-product-compliance
Ingram Content Group UK Ltd.
Pitfield, Milton Keynes, MK11 3LW, UK
UKHW041625031026
15587UKWH00001B/80

9 781498 548113